FREE Study Skills DVD Offer

Dear Customer,

Thank you for your purchase from Mometrix! We consider it an honor and a privilege that you have purchased our product and we want to ensure your satisfaction.

As a way of showing our appreciation and to help us better serve you, we have developed a Study Skills DVD that we would like to give you for FREE. This DVD covers our *best practices* for getting ready for your exam, from how to use our study materials to how to best prepare for the day of the test.

All that we ask is that you email us with feedback that would describe your experience so far with our product. Good, bad, or indifferent, we want to know what you think!

To get your FREE Study Skills DVD, email freedvd@mometrix.com with *FREE STUDY SKILLS DVD* in the subject line and the following information in the body of the email:

- The name of the product you purchased.
- Your product rating on a scale of 1-5, with 5 being the highest rating.
- Your feedback. It can be long, short, or anything in between. We just want to know your impressions and experience so far with our product. (Good feedback might include how our study material met your needs and ways we might be able to make it even better. You could highlight features that you found helpful or features that you think we should add.)
- Your full name and shipping address where you would like us to send your free DVD.

If you have any questions or concerns, please don't hesitate to contact me directly.

Thanks again!

Sincerely,

Jay Willis
Vice President
jay.willis@mometrix.com
1-800-673-8175

AF854991

NCMHCE
Practice Questions

NCMHCE Practice Tests and Exam Review for the National Clinical Mental Health Counseling Examination

Mometrix
TEST PREPARATION

Written and edited by Mometrix Test Prep

Printed in the United States of America

This paper meets the requirements of ANSI/NISO Z39.48-1992 (Permanence of Paper).

ISBN 13: 978-1-5167-3196-1
ISBN 10: 1-5167-3196-4

DEAR FUTURE EXAM SUCCESS STORY

First of all, **THANK YOU** for purchasing Mometrix study materials!

Second, congratulations! You are one of the few determined test-takers who are committed to doing whatever it takes to excel on your exam. **You have come to the right place.** We developed these practice tests with one goal in mind: to deliver you the best possible approximation of the questions you will see on test day.

Standardized testing is one of the biggest obstacles on your road to success, which only increases the importance of doing well in the high-pressure, high-stakes environment of test day. Your results on this test could have a significant impact on your future, and these practice tests will give you the repetitions you need to build your familiarity and confidence with the test content and format to help you achieve your full potential on test day.

Your success is our success

We would love to hear from you! If you would like to share the story of your exam success or if you have any questions or comments in regard to our products, please contact us at **800-673-8175** or **support@mometrix.com**.

Thanks again for your business and we wish you continued success!

Sincerely,
The Mometrix Test Preparation Team

Written and edited by Mometrix Test Prep
Printed in the United States of America

TABLE OF CONTENTS

Practice Test

Instructions

You have an examination booklet that contains ten simulations. Each simulation starts with a paragraph that gives preliminary information about a patient/client. The sections which follow are identified with a capital letter. Each section begins with specific instructions about the number of responses to select. You will indicate your selection, or selections, by placing a mark in the square. After you make your selection or selections, you will want to check your answers on the following page. The answer explanations and "Response Development" sections can provide insight and possibly additional information helpful in completing the other sections.

"Information Gathering" sections generally instruct you to "**select as many as you consider indicated.**" Read all of the choices before you select the responses you consider appropriate at that time for the patient/client.

"Decision Making" sections generally instruct you to "**select the most appropriate.**" Read all of the choices and then select the response you believe is the best.

This page is intentionally blank.

Simulation #1

Annette, an 18-year-old female is brought to your office by her parents. She is the eldest of three children. They note that she has been having marked difficulty with insomnia following the start of her new summertime swing-shift job (of about six weeks) as a clerk at a convenience store. She works from 4:00 p.m. until 1:00 a.m., Wednesday through Sunday, arriving home around 2:00 a.m., after the cash register check at shift change and the drive home. She has not been sleeping well; her appetite has been decreasing; and she seems uninterested in doing anything with her friends, with whom she used to be very socially active. As an aside, they also mention that she recently broke up with her boyfriend of two years just after she started the job.

NOW GO TO SECTION A.

Section A: Initial Information Gathering

Which of the following elements would be important in determining a presenting diagnosis? After making your selections and scoring your answers, it is beneficial to read the rationales and extended scenarios for all answer choices.

DIRECTIONS: Select as many as you consider indicated in this section.

- ☐ 1. Current stressors.
- ☐ 2. Educational history.
- ☐ 3. Quality of existing family relationships.
- ☐ 4. Mental status examination.
- ☐ 5. Appetite changes and eating patterns.
- ☐ 6. Family mental health history.
- ☐ 7. Insomnia persistence and patterns.
- ☐ 8. Depressive symptoms.
- ☐ 9. Current level of functioning.
- ☐ 10. Employment history.
- ☐ 11. Prior and/or current substances of abuse.
- ☐ 12. Client psychiatric history.

NOW GO TO SECTION B.

Section A: Relevance and Initial Information Explored

1. Current stressors
INDICATED (+2)

Currently living at home with parents. Apparently adequate social supports (family and friends). Recent break-up with a boyfriend of two years. The client becomes tearful and voices considerable distress at this loss, as she felt the relationship had been progressing well until recently.

2. Educational history
NOT INDICATED (-1)

No educational issues identified. High school graduate, reasonable grades, with appropriate developmental and intellectual functioning. Plans college in the fall.

3. Quality of existing family relationships.
INDICATED (+1)

The client was brought in by her parents, who voice genuine concern for her welfare. However, the client voices some tension between the parents and herself due to their pressuring her to find summer employment.

4. Mental status examination.
NOT INDICATED (-1)

No issues of cognitive impairment, bizarre behavior, suicidal ideation, etc., requiring address. Upon presentation, and in discussion with both the client and her parents, the client evidences a normal fund of information, appropriate verbal fluency, and reports full functional capacity in her employment.

5. Appetite changes and eating patterns.
INDICATED (+2)

Due to recent changes, appetite and eating patterns should be addressed. The client reports loss of interest in food, leading to an unintended weight loss of approximately 5 lbs. over the past month. By presentation, she does not appear either over- or underweight. However, she reports some sense that she is "heavy," and refers to the need for a "beach body, like some of my friends."

6. Family mental health history.
INDICATED (+1)

Any familial psychiatric history could bear upon the client's current situation. However, there is no reported family history of mental illness.

7. Insomnia persistence and patterns.
INDICATED (+3)

This was the chief complaint (by parents) at the time of presentation. Therefore, client's patterns of insomnia (delays in getting to sleep, returning to sleep, awakening too early, etc.) must be addressed—particularly as/if related to her new swing-shift work, and/or to depressive symptoms. The client reports difficulty getting adequate rest due to a variety of factors, including: 1) noise levels in the home; 2) distress over new adult life pressures (principally, full-time employment); 3) despair over the loss of her boyfriend; and 4) negative and discouraging thoughts intruding upon her thinking. Due to these manifold factors, the client primarily has difficulty getting to sleep, though staying asleep, and returning to sleep are also problematic.

8. Depressive symptoms.

INDICATED (+2)

The client exhibits multiple symptoms of depression, including: 1) dwelling on feelings of rejection, leading her to "feel down" and unwanted—mainly due to the boyfriend breaking off their relationship; 2) anhedonia (avoiding past friends and recreational activities, and spending exorbitant time alone in her bedroom); 3) tearfulness when discussing her feelings, especially the loss of her boyfriend and reduced social life due to summer work; 4) loss of appetite, and unintended weight loss of approximately 5 lbs.; and 5) restlessness and persistent insomnia due largely to intrusive and pressured thoughts of a negative and preoccupying nature.

9. Current level of functioning.

NOT INDICATED (-1)

All indications are that her baseline level of function is high. She is able to adhere to an employment schedule, functions well as a cashier, manages driving, and completes other responsible activities.

10. Employment history.

NOT INDICATED (-1)

The client's past employment has involved babysitting, house cleaning, and other age-appropriate jobs. She has not previously been discharged from, nor has she declined, any employment opportunity, per both the client and her parents.

11. Prior/current substances of abuse.

NOT INDICATED (-1)

The client has no past or current substance abuse.

12. Client psychiatric history.

INDICATED (+1)

The client has no other known history of a psychiatric nature, including no apparent history of depression or any history of psychiatric treatment or medications.

RESPONSE DEVELOPMENT:

The chief complaint at initial contact is that of insomnia (per the parents). The client is also struggling with: 1) a new job, leading to disruption in typical sleep periods; 2) stressors accompanying new entry into a full-time adult working role; 3) loss of appetite and interest in other previously important social and recreational pursuits; and, 4) the loss of an important romantic relationship of two years. Symptoms of depression are evident, including vegetative symptoms (e.g., anorexia, insomnia, anhedonia, tearfulness, etc.) and feelings of rejection and isolation. The differential diagnostic evaluation requires one to rule out: 1) major depression; 2) anorexia; 3) adjustment disorder with depressed mood; and 4) Circadian Rhythm Sleep Disorder.

This page is intentionally blank.

Section B: Based on the intake data, identify potential issues that need to be further addressed.

DIRECTIONS: Select as many as seem correct and necessary. After making your selections and scoring your answers, it is beneficial to read the rationales and extended scenarios for all answer choices.

- ☐ 1. Employment issues.
- ☐ 2. Family relationship issues.
- ☐ 3. Client's insight into coping.
- ☐ 4. Current symptoms of depression.
- ☐ 5. Substance abuse issues.
- ☐ 6. Sibling relationships in the home.

NOW GO TO SECTION C.

Section B: Relevance of Potential Information Needing Address:

1. Employment issues.
NOT INDICATED (-1)

The client is currently in a stable summer employment situation. Issues of her feelings about employment should be addressed with family relationship concerns, as related employment pressures were generated by her parents.

2. Family relationship issues.
INDICATED (+2)

The client expresses feelings of pressure to work, and her parents seem somewhat dismissive of her feelings about the loss of her boyfriend of two years.

3. Client's insight into coping.
INDICATED (+2)

The client is described as tearful and distressed over the loss of her boyfriend of two years. She also admits to feeling pressure and stress at her new full-time employment. She seems to lack adequate coping skills for her current situation.

4. Current symptoms of depression.
INDICATED (+3)

Symptoms of depression are evident, including vegetative symptoms (e.g., anorexia, insomnia, anhedonia, tearfulness, etc.) and feelings of rejection and isolation.

5. Substance abuse issues.
NOT INDICATED (-2)

There are no identified substance abuse issues.

6. Sibling relationships in the home.
NOT INDICATED (-3)

No sibling relationship issues have been raised.

Section C: Additional Information Gathering

What items among of the additional following would be most important in confirming an initial diagnosis?

DIRECTIONS: Select as many as you consider indicated in this Section. After making your selections and scoring your answers, it is beneficial to read the rationales and extended scenarios for all answer choices.

- ☐ 1. The Beck Depression Inventory-II.
- ☐ 2. Seasonal mood patterns.
- ☐ 3. Weight changes.
- ☐ 4. Medical history.
- ☐ 5. Women's Health Initiative Insomnia Rating Scale (WHI-IRS).
- ☐ 6. Traumatic life events.
- ☐ 7. Social history.
- ☐ 8. Educational achievement.
- ☐ 9. Suicidal Ideation.
- ☐ 10. Religious affiliation/attendance.
- ☐ 11. Legal issues.
- ☐ 12. Financial issues.

NOW GO TO SECTION D.

Section C: Element Relevance and Secondary Information Obtained

1. The Beck Depression Inventory-II.
INDICATED (+2)

The client demonstrates multiple symptoms of depression (e.g., anorexia, insomnia, anhedonia, tearfulness, feelings of rejection and isolation) and therefore, use of this instrument is indicated. The Beck Depression Inventory-II assists in the identification of depression. A total score of 0-13 is considered minimal range, 14-19 is mild, 20-28 is moderate, and 29-63 is severe. The client scored 22.

2. Seasonal mood patterns.
NOT INDICATED (-1)

Although the client's presentation is related to issues of mood, there is nothing to suggest Depressive Disorder with Seasonal Pattern. The client's issues of depression appear to be related to situational circumstances, rather than to a seasonally based pattern of mood changes.

3. Weight changes.
INDICATED (+1)

The client has experienced unintended weight loss, and thus, issues of eating and appetite must be explored. While the client does acknowledge "body image" issues, she denies any intentional effort to restrict her caloric intake at this time. Further, she specifically denies any binging and purging patterns that would be characteristic of bulimia.

4. Medical history.
INDICATED (+1)

The parents report that the client was seen by her primary care physician within the last week. No medical problems were identified.

5. Women's Health Initiative Insomnia Rating Scale (WHI-IRS).
INDICATED (+3)

Both the client and her parents acknowledge that insomnia is a problem (with sleep averaging 6 hours or less each night). The client indicates problem onset at one week after she began her shift work, right about the time her boyfriend broke off their relationship. The client's primary sleep problem is an inability to fall asleep, although other sleep disturbances do occur (including being awakened by noise in the home during her sleep hours). The WHI-IRS score can be calculated as the average of scores for trouble falling asleep, waking several times, waking early, trouble resuming sleep, and overall sleep quality. Scores ≥ 9 (range: 0-20) indicate clinically significant insomnia. The client scored 11.

6. Traumatic Life events.
NOT INDICATED (-1)

No traumatic life events have been identified.

7. Social history.

INDICATED (+2)

The client recently graduated from high school. She has a number of friends, but is not able to spend time with most of them due to the hours she works. Thus, feelings of isolation and social estrangement are particularly acute at this time. However, the parents also report that the friends do call and invite her to join them during her days off and/or hours when she is not working, but the client declines these offers. The client acknowledges this, but explains that her boyfriend normally accompanied her to social events, and feels that it will be awkward showing up at social events newly alone.

8. Educational achievement.

NOT INDICATED (-1)

No issues of an educational nature have been raised.

9. Suicidal ideation.

INDICATED (+1)

Given the client's symptoms of depression, questioning regarding suicidal ideation is reasonably indicated. The client denies any thoughts, intent, or plans to self-harm in any way.

10. Religious affiliation/attendance.

NOT INDICATED (-1)

No issues related to religion have been raised.

11. Legal issues.

NOT INDICATED (-1)

No legal issues have been identified.

12. Financial issues.

NOT INDICATED (-1)

The client lives with her parents in an apparently stable home situation. Summer work is purportedly for her to contribute meaningfully to her college education, and not because her parents are not able to afford to assist her.

RESPONSE DEVELOPMENT:

The client is an 18-year-old, living with parents, with new adult responsibilities (full-time summer work), the recent loss of a significant two-year relationship, and ongoing estrangement from friends and recreational activities due to swing-shift work hours, including all weekends. She is also avoiding social contacts with friends when she is available, due to recent break up with boyfriend, who moved in the same social circles as the client. Complains of insomnia, purportedly due to swing-shift sleep disruption and sleep hours disturbed by in-home activities during her sleep hours. Evidences symptoms of depression, including vegetative symptoms (e.g., anorexia with 5 lbs. unintentional weight loss, insomnia, anhedonia, tearfulness, etc.) and feelings of rejection and isolation. Has positive scores for depression on the Beck Depression Inventory-II, and for insomnia on the Women's Health Initiative – Insomnia Rating Scale (WHI-IRS).

This page is intentionally blank.

Section D: Provisional Diagnosis Formulation

Based upon the available information, what would appear to be the most appropriate provisional diagnosis?

DIRECTIONS: Select the most appropriate primary diagnosis indicated in this Section. Check your answer. If your answer is not the one indicated write down your point value, then choose another answer and check your score again. Your score from this section will be the numbers added together. (For example: If your first choice was not indicated and had a score of -1, and your second answer choice was the one indicated with a score of +3, your score for this section would be a +2.)

- ☐ 1. Circadian Rhythm Sleep Disorder - Shift Work Type (G47.26).
- ☐ 2. Bereavement, assumed death of family member (Z63.4).
- ☐ 3. Major Depressive Disorder, Single Episode, Mild (F32.0).
- ☐ 4. Adjustment Disorder, With Depressed Mood (F43.21).
- ☐ 5. Other Depressive Episodes (F32.8).
- ☐ 6. Insomnia, unspecified (G47.00).

NOW GO TO SECTION E.

Section D: Relevance and Diagnostic Formulation.

1. Circadian Rhythm Sleep Disorder - Shift Work Type (G47.26).
NOT INDICATED (-1)

DSM criteria indicate that the "pattern of sleep disruption" must be due primarily to "a mismatch between the sleep-wake schedule required by a person's environment and his or her circadian [or natural] sleep-wake pattern." This client, however, describes stressful life issues leading to intrusive and distressing thoughts that keep her awake. Further, this diagnosis would not be made when sleep disturbance occurs "exclusively during the course of another...mental disorder." Given that the client's problems began one week after she started her job, and right at the time of her break-up with her boyfriend, better diagnostic options exist.

2. Bereavement, assumed death of family member (Z63.4).
NOT INDICATED (-2)

Although an issue of "loss" is involved (i.e., the loss of a significant two-year relationship), this category of bereavement is intended to be applied only in situations of loss due to death.

3. Major Depressive Disorder, Single Episode, Mild (F32.0).
NOT INDICATED (-1)

The client does indeed have significant symptoms of depression. These include anorexia, insomnia, anhedonia, tearfulness, etc. However, the "major" depressive category is generally intended for characteristics more severe than those indicated here. For example, the client's weight does not exceed 5% of total weight; issues of fatigue, poor concentration, psychomotor agitation, and suicidal ideation are also not adequately present. Further, there appears to be a primary precipitant to her melancholia—specifically, the loss of her boyfriend. In addition, numerous other very transient factors seem to be influencing and sustaining the course of her depression—e.g., transitioning to adulthood; coping with a first full-time job; separation from friends and loss of routine recreational opportunities, etc. Consequently, this diagnostic category does not appear to be appropriate.

4. Adjustment Disorder, With Depressed Mood (F43.21).
INDICATED (+3)

Correct Selection. The emotional (depressive) symptoms are "in response" to clearly identifiable situational factors. The diagnosis also allows for multiple "stressors" to be involved. The symptoms must have onset "within 3 months of the onset of the stressors," and these symptoms began within a week or so. The requisite "marked distress that is in excess of what would be expected" and "significant impairment in social" functioning is in evidence. It is also reasonable to expect that, with proper support, the symptoms will "not persist for more than an additional 6 months." This would be the most accurate working diagnosis available, given the information provided.

5. Other Depressive Episodes (F32.8).
NOT INDICATED (-1)

Depressive symptoms are amply in evidence. Further, there are a number of potential precipitants to the depression that impede the diagnostic process—swing-shift work and related insomnia; isolation from friends; loss of a romantic relationship; problems adjusting to adult life; etc. However, there is sufficient clinical information available for a more accurate diagnosis, beyond

"Depressive Disorder Not Otherwise Specified." Where such information is in evidence, it is incumbent upon the clinician to make a more targeted diagnosis.

6. Insomnia, unspecified (G47.00).

NOT INDICATED (-1)

This is not the best option, as in the criteria for insomnia it states that there cannot be coexisting medical or mental disorders that could cause the insomnia. Though the patient has a positive score for insomnia, there are several clear reasons for the client's insomnia and/or sleep disturbance.

This page is intentionally blank.

Section E: Based on the provisional diagnosis, what treatment methods and referrals would be appropriate for Annette, the client?

DIRECTIONS: Select as many as you consider indicated in this Section. After making your selections and scoring your answers, it is beneficial to read the rationales and extended scenarios for all answer choices.

- ☐ 1. Psychiatrist Referral to Evaluate Medication Needs.
- ☐ 2. Family Counseling.
- ☐ 3. Participation in a young adult support group.
- ☐ 4. Stress Management Counseling.
- ☐ 5. Illness Insight Counseling.
- ☐ 6. Psychoanalysis.
- ☐ 7. Medications Compliance Monitoring and Counseling.
- ☐ 8. Cognitive Behavioral Therapy.
- ☐ 9. Individual counseling.

NOW GO TO SECTION F.

Section E: Treatment Approach Relevance and Selection.

1. Psychiatrist Referral to Evaluate Medication Needs.
NOT INDICATED (-1)

Medications to address the client's depression may eventually be required (especially if the adjustment process unfolds with difficulty and the client evolves into a Major Depression). However, at this juncture the client at least needs further evaluation and treatment initiation before this decision is made.

2. Family Counseling.
INDICATED (+2)

Incongruence between the client's and the parents' goals seems to be in evidence—specifically, the need for full-time employment throughout this first summer, and especially in the face of the loss of a two-year relationship. At this juncture, it appears that the client's coping skills are inadequate to properly cope with the sudden nature of these demands.

3. Participation in a young adult support group.
INDICATED (+1)

The client's situation suggests that she may yet benefit from a group experience. However, the greatest benefit will most likely be realized after adequate progress has been made in individual counseling sessions.

4. Stress Management Counseling.
INDICATED (+2)

The client obviously lacks the coping skills to cope with the new stressors in her life. Therefore, this approach may be useful in conjunction with grief counseling.

5. Illness-specific Insight Counseling.
NOT INDICATED (-2)

The client is not suffering from any illness requiring counseling of this nature.

6. Psychoanalysis.
NOT INDICATED (-2)

The long-term nature of this therapeutic approach makes it ill-suited to effectively address the client's current issues.

7. Medications Compliance Monitoring and Counseling.
NOT INDICATED (-2)

The client has not yet been provided any medications, and therefore, counseling of this nature is not required.

8. Cognitive-Behavioral Therapy.
NOT INDICATED (-1)

This technique is most useful in situations where understanding and behavioral change are required. In this situation, a counseling approach of this nature would not be among the most effective approaches available.

9. Individual Counseling.
INDICATED (+2)

It is highly likely that this client will benefit from an individual counseling approach, as it will allow for a more personalized intervention, as well as the establishment of a therapeutic alliance and trust necessary for coping with her current stressors.

This page is intentionally blank.

Section F: Based on the selected treatment modalities, what information and monitoring methods would be appropriate for Annette, the client?

DIRECTIONS: Select as many as you consider indicated in this section. After making your selections and scoring your answers, it is beneficial to read the rationales and extended scenarios for all answer choices.

- ☐ 1. Progress notes in the counseling record.
- ☐ 2. Substance abuse monitoring.
- ☐ 3. Medications monitoring.
- ☐ 4. Affective functioning.
- ☐ 5. Social interactions.
- ☐ 6. Mood graph.
- ☐ 7. Energy level.
- ☐ 8. Cognitive functioning.

NOW GO TO SECTION G.

Section F: Information and Monitoring Methods.

1. Progress notes in the counseling record.
INDICATED (+2)

Clinician entries in the client's counseling record can be an excellent way to monitor the interventions used and the client's subsequent progress.

2. Substance Abuse Monitoring.
NOT INDICATED (-2)

There are no issues of substance abuse, and thus, this monitoring would not be indicated.

3. Medication Monitoring.
NOT INDICATED (-2)

The client has not been prescribed any medications. Therefore, this monitoring would not be indicated.

4. Affective Functioning
INDICATED (+1)

Any further deterioration in the client's status should readily become apparent in the client's affective presentation. Therefore, this should be followed closely.

5. Social Interactions
INDICATED (+1)

The client has been socially isolated, due to work and stressors related to the loss of a boyfriend with whom she routinely attended social events. Careful monitoring of social interactions can aid in determining the client's rate of reintroduction into her social affairs, as well as any further deterioration in this important index of recovery.

6. Mood Graph.
INDICATED (+2)

The use of a Mood Graph for the client and the clinician to mutually track the client's changes in mood, and any progress or deterioration over time, would be very helpful in this situation.

7. Energy Level.
INDICATED (+1)

Listlessness, fatigue, and other indices of psychomotor retardation can signal a deterioration in the client's condition, and therefore, should be followed closely.

8. Cognitive Functioning.
NOT INDICATED (-2)

All current reports indicate that the client's cognitive functioning is fully adequate and within normal parameters. Therefore, monitoring of this nature does not appear to be necessary at this time. Only if the client's depression progresses, such that increased distractibility, forgetfulness, and reduced attention span are noted, would cognitive functioning be further considered.

This page is intentionally blank.

Section G: In developing a collaborative treatment plan with the client, what items among the following should be included?

DIRECTIONS: Select as many as you consider indicated in this section. After making your selections and scoring your answers, it is beneficial to read the rationales and extended scenarios for all answer choices.

- ☐ 1. Jointly identify appropriate treatment goals.
- ☐ 2. Complete information release forms for future needs.
- ☐ 3. Develop the specific objectives to meet the identified goals.
- ☐ 4. Produce a suicide contract to ensure client safety.
- ☐ 5. Discuss the issue of confidentiality.

Section G: Treatment Plan Development Options - Relevance and Selection.

1. Jointly identify appropriate treatment goals.
INDICATED (+2)

Client buy-in to the treatment process and progress toward desired outcomes will typically be enhanced when the establishment of treatment goals is shared between the client and clinician.

2. Complete information release forms for future needs.
NOT INDICATED (-2)

Information release forms are completed only in circumstances of clear need. They must have explicit identification of the party(ies) to whom the information is being released, the specific purpose(s), and an expiration date. Such criteria cannot be formulated in advance of need.

3. Develop the specific objectives to meet the identified goals.
INDICATED (+2)

Identification of the steps to goal achievement deepens client commitment and overall clarity of necessary steps and expectations.

4. Produce a suicide contract to ensure client safety.
NOT INDICATED (-1)

The client has specifically denied any suicidal ideation or intent. Therefore, "contracting" around the issue of suicidality would be premature (and would likely not ever be needed, given the client's current level of cooperation—e.g., answers questions with detail and honesty, etc.).

5. Discuss the issue of confidentiality.
INDICATED (+1)

Every client needs to know the scope and limits of confidentiality in the context of counseling, and it should be addressed at the outset of the counseling experience.

SCORING: (Max = maximum possible; MPL = minimum passing level)

1A. Max 12; MPL 8
1B. Max 7; MPL 5
1C. Max 10; MPL 7
1D. Max 3; MPL 2
1E. Max 7; MPL 5
1F. Max 7; MPL 5
1G. Max 5; MPL 4

Simulation #2

You are an outside-contract forensic counselor for a locked state hospital. You are called to evaluate a 61-year-old widowed Southeast Asian (Laotian) male for his capacity to stand trial. He speaks no English, but a skilled interpreter is made available to you. The patient was arrested for a charge of indecent exposure ("flashing" a passerby in a shopping mall lingerie outlet). At the time of his arrest, his family acknowledged that he has episodically engaged in this behavior at various times over the past several years. The current arrest was for a flagrant episode of conduct, witnessed by numerous persons, and therefore, no questions of actual intent remain. However, due to questions about culture, the language barrier, and the patient's reluctance to discuss anything with legal staff (including his public defender), competency to stand trial could not be adequately ascertained. Thus, he was remanded by the courts into the state facility for further psychiatric evaluation. You are to provide that evaluation.

NOW GO TO SECTION A.

Section A: Initial Information Gathering.

Based upon the information provided, what items among the following elements would be important in initially evaluating the client and formulating a provisional diagnosis?

DIRECTIONS: Select as many as you consider correct. After making your selections and scoring your answers, it is beneficial to read the rationales and extended scenarios for all answer choices.

- ☐ 1. Mental status screening.
- ☐ 2. Residential history.
- ☐ 3. Medical history.
- ☐ 4. Educational history.
- ☐ 5. Psychosexual cultural norms.
- ☐ 6. Psychiatric history.
- ☐ 7. Substance abuse history.
- ☐ 8. Mood status.
- ☐ 9. Vocational/employment history.
- ☐ 10. Legal history.

NOW GO TO SECTION B.

Section A: Relevance and Initial Information Obtained.

1. Mental Status Screening.
INDICATED (+2)

The patient refused to cooperate in a formal mini-mental status examination (the standardized Folstein), but an abbreviated exam was completed by simply talking with him. In this manner, the client was found to be an oriented person (name, date of birth, age, etc.), as well as to year, season, month, calendar date, day of the week, country, state, city, facility name, unit name, and room number—a perfect score of 10 out of 10 for orientation. While the client declined to perform serial calculations, he was readily able to calculate how many years it had been since he was married, living in his homeland, living in the United States, widowed, etc. He was also able to write out and correctly spell the names of various places in his homeland, to properly recall the time our session began and was expected to end (as told at the outset)—resulting in an abbreviated Registration/ Calculation/ Memory score of 11 out of 11. Finally, he scored 3 of 3 in the language, object naming, and communication measures provided. The result was an abbreviated score of 24 out of 24 (as opposed to the usual MMSE upper maximum score of 30)—absent only short-term memory testing and the following of multiple staged commands. Consequently, the client appeared to be without any obvious cognitive deficits at the time of this contact.

2. Residential History.
NOT INDICATED (-1)

Although information about the patient's residential history is meaningful, it would not be relevant to the formulation of a diagnosis. Even so, the client was born and raised in Laos. He was conscripted into the military in his late teens, but left that country after the death of his wife (in the war) and after the country fell into communist hands. He then fled to Thailand, where he lived for several years in refugee camps. Finally, he was brought to the United States nine years previously through a refugee relocation program. It was here that the behaviors of concern apparently first began.

3. Medical History.
INDICATED (+1)

The patient denied any history of head trauma, neurological disorders, endocrine (including thyroid) disorders, and no metabolic issues, etc.—to the degree he understood these medical problems. The patient is a chronic 1-pack-per day smoker, and typically drank (beer) recreationally prior to his arrest and incarceration.

4. Educational History.
NOT INDICATED (-1)

Not relevant to formulating a DSM diagnosis. However, the patient was only able to complete the equivalent of an approximately 4th grade education in his native land. This was sufficient, however, for him to be able to read and write adequately in his native language (Laotian).

5. Psychosexual Cultural Norms.
INDICATED (+2)

In consultation with both the patient and the Laotian interpreter it was determined that standards of modesty and sexual propriety in the patient's native land and culture are similar to those found in the United States. Therefore, the conduct with which he was charged in this country would be seen in a similar light in his homeland.

6. Psychiatric History.
INDICATED (+2)

The patient has a history of combat military service. His spouse was also killed during that time. Further exploration indicates that the patient has a likely past history of PTSD-like symptoms, which apparently resolved during the ensuing years. Beyond this, the patient has no known psychiatric history, hospitalizations, medications, or any prior treatment.

7. Substance abuse.
INDICATED (+2)

The patient admits to a very remote history of rare opium use (smoking), but denies any current use.

8. Mood Status.
INDICATED (+1)

The patient presented as quite depressed, affectively restricted, and episodically tearful.

9. Vocational/employment.
NOT INDICATED (-2)

Not germane to the diagnostic process. Even so, the patient has no special skills or training. He worked as a rice farmer when younger, and then spent much of his adult life in the military, with only foot-soldier combat training. For a few years prior to fleeing his country, he worked for a Laotian metropolitan airport as a baggage handler.

10. Legal History.
INDICATED (+1)

The patient has no known prior legal history. He was arrested some four weeks previously, and remained in jail during an initial evaluation period. He was seen by jail psychiatry staff only for evaluation for possible suicidal ideation, and was psychiatry cleared at that time. It is unclear from the record how this determination was made, as the record only reports the referral and the cursory findings (again via an interpreter).

RESPONSE DEVELOPMENT:

The patient is a 61-year-old widowed male refugee from Laos, arrested on charges of indecent exposure. He presents as cognitively intact (per MMSE), but often uncooperative with the evaluation process. He has a history of past military combat trauma, possible PTSD (resolved), and has suffered the war-based death of his wife, dislocation from his native land, and two subsequently major relocations (Thailand and the United States). There appears to be no cultural psychosexual basis for his behavior. Some evidence of depression, but this would be a generally normal response to his situation.

This page is intentionally blank.

Section B: Based on the intake data, identify areas needing further evaluation.

DIRECTIONS: Select as many as seem correct and necessary. After making your selections and scoring your answers, it is beneficial to read the rationales and extended scenarios for all answer choices.

- ☐ 1. Support Systems.
- ☐ 2. Suicidality.
- ☐ 3. Stress management.
- ☐ 4. Communication issues.
- ☐ 5. Educational issues.
- ☐ 6. Impulse control.
- ☐ 7. Employment issues.
- ☐ 8. Substance abuse issues.

NOW GO TO SECTION C.

Section B: Relevance of Potential Information Needing Address and Findings.

1. Support Systems.
INDICATED (+1)

Given his circumstances and obvious depressive affect, the patient could benefit from further social support. Contact with extended relatives (adult siblings, adult nieces and nephews) reveals that they are extremely embarrassed over what has occurred, while willing to offer distant support (minimal financial assistance for non-legal immediate personal needs, and receiving occasional telephone calls). However, most are located at some distance from the treating facility, and none are willing to become intensely involved in his personal situation.

2. Suicidality.
INDICATED (+1)

There is some affective indication of depression, and as the patient's situation becomes clearer to him, his depression could worsen. Therefore, exploring any suicidal ideation would be important. In talking with the patient further, he denies any intent or plan for self-harm, and agrees to openly discuss such feelings if they arise.

3. Stress Management.
INDICATED (+2)

The patient is in an obviously stressful situation. In further discussion, the patient reveals additional stressors, including estrangement from his family, shame over his conduct, fear about the legal system, etc.

4. Communication Issues.
INDICATED (+1)

The language barrier and related cultural issues have been significant. Further exploration with the patient reveals additional sociocultural stress related to the use of an interpreter. The individual was contracted by the facility through a local Southeast Asian resource center. He is a young college student who is an ethnic Indochinese Mien individual, fluent in Laotian, Hmong, and Mien. Given his multilingual skills, he is an ideal candidate for working at the center. However, socioculturally, many Laotians see themselves as more advanced and otherwise superior to both of these other ethnic groups. Therefore, the patient feels reluctant to communicate openly through this individual—particularly about the charges pending against him. Finally, the interpreter is very young, and coming from an age-conscious Asian society, the situation of dependency on one so young is further distressing to the patient.

5. Educational issues.
NOT INDICATED (-1)

There are no relevant educational issues identified for this older Southeast Asian patient.

6. Impulse control.
INDICATED (+2)

By reports and presentation, the client appears to have poor impulse control. In further discussion, the client finally admits to his behavior and emphasizes the fact that he had acted on impulse.

However, he minimizes the nature of his recent conduct (suggests his exposure was very limited), and emphatically denies any prior history of such behavior—even when confronted with the fact that his family states otherwise.

7. Employment issues.
NOT INDICATED (-1)

The patient has been receiving welfare and Medicaid benefits over the last nine years, which are expected to continue. There are no employment issues requiring further address.

8. Substance Abuse Issues.
NOT INDICATED (-1)

All available information suggests that there are no current substance abuse issues that need to be addressed.

This page is intentionally blank.

Section C: Additional Information Gathering.

Over the next several weeks, you continue to interact with this patient on a regular basis. As he becomes acclimated to the facility and its routine, his depressive symptoms subside, he becomes much more interactive with other patients, and his attitude toward you begins to evolve. He moves from being very pliant and responsive to your efforts to engage him, to being increasingly resistant and non-compliant. The time comes when, upon seeing you, he turns his back and attempts to ignore you. Still later, when he sees you approaching, he takes to smiling deceptively and then blatantly ignoring your efforts to meet with him. Looking directly at you, he turns to engage others and walks away even when you're speaking to him. In consultation with other staff, you discover that he has been given various language-independent (image- and manipulative-based) psychiatric examinations, and has been routinely failing them all. Staff are uncertain what is happening, but are inclined to conclude that he is indeed not competent to stand trial.

To better determine the client's level of function, cognitive capacity, and current behavioral presentation, what additional data may be helpful?

DIRECTIONS: Select the most appropriate options provided in this section. After making your selections and scoring your answers, it is beneficial to read the rationales and extended scenarios for all answer choices.

- ☐ 1. Direct interviews with the patient's daily attending staff.
- ☐ 2. Staff psychiatry contacts and records review.
- ☐ 3. Medical records review.
- ☐ 4. Collateral contact with the patient's family.
- ☐ 5. Substance abuse testing review.
- ☐ 6. Updated legal review.

NOW GO TO SECTION D.

Section C: Additional Information Gathering and Findings.

1. Direct interviews with the patient's daily attending staff.
INDICATED (+2)

The daily attending staff can address the patient's capacity to function in numerous ways: 1) tidiness; 2) appropriate daily dressing; 3) capacity to showing up for meals as well as selection of food and eating habits; 4) hygiene and grooming performance; and 5) daily behavioral patterns with staff and other facility patients. Subsequent interviews indicate that the patient maintains a well-ordered room, dresses properly and without prompts, and shows up for meals and activities without supervision (and often uses gestures, etc., to ensure he knows where he should be and when). He also bathes and seeks clean clothing and bedding readily, and interacts easily and comfortably with other facility patients—indeed, surprisingly well, given the language barrier.

2. Staff psychiatry contacts and records review.
INDICATED (+2)

Testing psychologists express concern about the patient's capacity, both during your interview and in the written clinical record. During testing, the client is unable to match related pictures and objects, perseverates in drawing exercises, and seems generally confused and psychiatrically impaired.

3. Medical records review.
INDICATED (+1)

Subsequent medical testing has revealed no apparent organic deficits, biological dysfunction, or other physiological impediment. Tests have included extensive blood testing to rule out biochemical imbalances and endocrinological diseases, as well as CT and MRI scans to rule out stroke, brain tumors, hydrocephalus; and other cerebral impediments, and clinical neurological evaluation to determine if there are any other signs of neurological dysfunction. All testing has been negative, indicating the patient is otherwise healthy.

4. Collateral contact with the patient's family.
INDICATED (+1)

Follow-up contacts with the patient's extended family indicate that they are not aware of any problems with the patient as well. Much like attending facility staff, they have consistently found the patient to be free of any inappropriate thought distortions, bizarre behavior, confusion, and/or other symptoms of compromise. Quite the opposite, the patient speaks with them easily and cogently, remembers past conversations, and is quite normal and appropriate to their appraisal.

5. Substance Abuse Testing Review.
NOT INDICATED (-1)

The patient has no ongoing substance abuse issues. Further, he is in a locked treatment facility and thus, illicit substances of abuse would not be available to him.

6. Updated Legal Review.

INDICATED (+1)

Contact with the patient's public defender yields no further information. Review of the arresting record, jail psychiatry reports, and other available records indicates no signs of psychotic or otherwise bizarre behavior at the time of the patient's arrest.

RESPONSE DEVELOPMENT:

The patient has been medically cleared in all health domains, and facility support and allied healthcare staff report no problems with the patient of any kind. Indeed, both support staff and the patient's family indicate that the patient moves easily around the facility, maintains excellent self-care, shows up on time and where he should be for meals and activities, etc., and interacts easily and successfully with other patients, family, and ancillary care staff. While psychiatric testing suggests the patient may have various deficits, there seems reason to believe that the client's presentation with testing staff has been deliberately contrived. With this in mind, further review with psychiatric staff ensues. In one test, it was noted that the patient was unable to differentiate between a picture of a ball and an airplane. Given that the patient previously worked as a baggage handler at an airport, this would suggest gross decompensation on his part. To further engage the client, you remind him that you will soon be submitting a report to the courts, at which point he consents to meet with you. On the way from his room, however, he pauses to pull on a dress shirt over his t-shirt (which he buttons properly), to pick up a comb (which he uses properly) as he follows you to a meeting room, and to complain that you're causing him to miss a haircut (and he asks you, via the interpreter, to delay your meeting to allow for it). Clearly, the patient is fully able to attend to dress, hygiene, grooming, appointments, etc.

Section D: Based on the information above, what provisional primary diagnosis would be appropriate for this client?

DIRECTIONS: Select the one most appropriate primary diagnosis. Check your answer. If your answer is not the one indicated write down your point value, then choose another answer and check your score again. Your score from this section will be the numbers added together. (For example: If your first choice was not indicated and had a score of -1, and your second answer choice was the one indicated with a score of +3, your score for this section would be a +2.)

- ☐ 1. Post-Traumatic Stress Disorder, unspecified (F43.10).
- ☐ 2. Exhibitionistic Disorder (F65.2).
- ☐ 3. Brief Psychotic Disorder (F23).
- ☐ 4. Frotteurism (F65.81).
- ☐ 5. Factitious Disorder (F68.1).
- ☐ 6. Adjustment Disorder with Depressed Mood (F43.21).

NOW GO TO SECTION E.

Section D: Diagnostic Review and Formulation.

1. Post-Traumatic Stress Disorder, unspecified (F43.10).
NOT INDICATED (-1)

All reports indicate that any symptoms of PTSD appear to have resolved long ago.

2. Exhibitionistic Disorder (F65.2).
NOT INDICATED (-1)

This would not be the most proximal (primary) diagnosis, as it is not the current focus of treatment/engagement at this juncture. However, it is the proper label for the client's arrest behavior. He meets criteria, as reports indicate the behavior is recurrent, and certainly for a period longer than the requisite six months.

3. Brief Psychotic Disorder (F23).
NOT INDICATED (-1)

The arresting report and reports from jail staff and psychiatry indicate that there was no apparent evidence of psychosis at the time of the patient's arrest and during his incarceration. Similarly, no evidence of psychosis has emerged since the patient's arrival at the state mental hospital.

4. Frotteurism (F65.81).
NOT INDICATED (-1)

The essential features of this diagnosis are touching and rubbing against others for sexual arousal. The patient has not demonstrated either of these features.

5. Factitious Disorder (F68.1).
INDICATED (+3)

All available evidence (excepting only brief episodes of psychiatric testing using pictures and/or manipulatives) indicates that this patient has been feigning psychiatric illness in order to evade further involvement with the courts, and to escape sentencing for his criminal behavior.

6. Adjustment Disorder with Depressed Mood (F43.21).
NOT INDICATED (-1)

The patient had evidence of depression early on in the evaluative process. Certainly, there were issues in adjustment following the processes of arrest and incarceration.

RESPONSE FORMATION

The current provisional DSM-5 diagnoses for this client would be:

1. Factitious Disorder (F68.1).
2. Exhibitionistic Disorder (F65.2).
3. Nicotine dependence, unspecified, uncomplicated (F17.200).

Section E: Based on the provisional diagnosis, what theoretical approach might work best for this client?

DIRECTIONS: Select the one most appropriate therapy. Check your answer. If your answer is not the one indicated write down your point value, then choose another answer and check your score again. Your score from this section will be the numbers added together.

- ☐ 1. Person-centered therapy.
- ☐ 2. Cognitive-behavioral therapy.
- ☐ 3. Freudian therapy.
- ☐ 4. Glasser's reality therapy.
- ☐ 5. Adlerian therapy.
- ☐ 6. Existential therapy.

Section E: Element Relevance and Commentary.

1. Person-Centered Therapy.
NOT INDICATED (-1)

This approach works well for situational disorders, self-esteem issues, etc., but it is less than ideal for a Factitious Disorder and Exhibitionistic Disorder.

2. Cognitive-Behavioral Therapy.
INDICATED (+3)

This approach is ideal for a Factitious Disorder. This approach, combined with medications, is also appropriate for the treatment of Exhibitionistic Disorder.

3. Freudian Therapy.
NOT INDICATED (-1)

This therapeutic approach is best suited to short-term interventions around depression and anxiety, and long-term therapy with dissociative disorders and personality disorders.

4. Glasser's Reality Therapy.
NOT INDICATED (-1)

This approach could be used with a patient with Factitious Disorder, but is less meaningful in the treatment of Exhibitionistic Disorder. Therefore, it would not be the first treatment option in this situation.

5. Adlerian Therapy.
NOT INDICATED (-1)

The Adlerian approach is well-suited to marital concerns, parent-child conflicts, acting out, and other emotive issues in otherwise healthy clients, but less so for the more serious Factitious Disorder and Exhibitionistic Disorder.

6. Existential Therapy.
NOT INDICATED (-1)

This approach works best for individuals coping with anxiety or depression, but is not ideal in situations of Factitious Disorder and Exhibitionistic Disorder.

SCORING: (Max = maximum possible; MPL = minimum passing level)

2A. Max 11; MPL 8
2B. Max 7; MPL 5
2C. Max 7; MPL 6
2D. Max 3; MPL 2
2E. Max 3; MPL 2

Simulation #3

Mark, a 25-year-old Caucasian male, calls for an appointment without disclosing any specific concerns. He works for a barber and beauty supply business, and drives a local delivery route in and around the city in which he resides. He has been married for two years, and he and his wife have one newborn child.

NOW GO TO SECTION A.

Section A: Initial Information Gathering.

The client seems reluctant to reveal his reason for seeking counseling. What might you do and say to put him more at ease?

DIRECTIONS: Select as many as you consider correct. After making your selections and scoring your answers, it is beneficial to read the rationales and extended scenarios for all answer choices.

- ☐ 1. Can you tell me what's on your mind?
- ☐ 2. Do you have any concerns about seeing a counselor?
- ☐ 3. Shall we discuss my fee schedule?
- ☐ 4. Who referred you to see me?
- ☐ 5. Most people seeing a counselor just need some feedback about their lives. What brings you in today?
- ☐ 6. Do you understand that homework may be required?

NOW GO TO SECTION B.

Section A: Element Relevance and Initial Information Obtained.

1. Can you tell me what's on your mind?
INDICATED (+2)

This question is open and non-threatening, and it allows the client to easily express his concerns in any way that suits him.

2. Do you have any concerns about seeing a counselor?
NOT INDICATED (-1)

While this is a forthright question, it presumes the client is worried about seeing the counselor, and may prompt a defensive (or overly reassuring) response.

3. Shall we discuss my fee schedule?
NOT INDICATED (-2)

This question could be seen as downright disrespectful and suggests that the client is either miserly or else unable to afford the counseling services.

4. Who referred you to see me?
NOT INDICATED (-2)

This question could be perceived as an attempt by the counselor to pursue marketing and referral concerns, instead of voicing genuine concern about the client and his reasons for being there.

5. Most people seeing a counselor just need some feedback about their lives. What brings you in today?
INDICATED: (+2)

This question "normalizes" the clinical engagement process, and then allows the client to frame a response in his own way.

6. Do you understand that homework may be required?
NOT INDICATED (-2)

This question suggests that the client is either lazy or resistant, or both. Therefore, it is not an appropriate intake question.

Section B: Identify the most positive client-therapist spatial arrangement in an office during an initial intake session:

DIRECTIONS: Select the arrangement likely to be helpful to the client at intake. After making your selections and scoring your answers, it is beneficial to read the rationales and extended scenarios for all answer choices.

- ☐ 1. The counselor and client seated at an angle from each other with nothing between them.
- ☐ 2. The counselor and client seated across a desk from each other.
- ☐ 3. The counselor seated directly in front of a diploma and certification plaques to reassure the client.
- ☐ 4. The counselor standing and pacing while talking to the client.
- ☐ 5. The client recumbent on a couch while talking with the counselor.

NOW GO TO SECTION C.

Section B: The value and relevance of potential information to share.

1. The counselor and client seated at an angle from each other with nothing between them.
MOST USEFUL (+3)

This spatial arrangement suggests equality, and an open engagement process.

2. The counselor and client seated across a desk from each other.
LESS USEFUL (+1)

This spatial arrangement suggests a professional barrier exists between the counselor and client.

3. The counselor seated directly in front of a diploma and certification plaques to reassure the client.
LESS USEFUL (-1)

This suggests either an attempt at professional dominance, or an effort to cover professional insecurity. Neither will benefit the encounter. While the presence of credentials can be appropriate, the placement should be non-threatening.

4. The counselor standing and pacing while talking to the client.
NOT USEFUL (-2)

Pacing in the presence of a client would be distracting, agitating, and suggest a marked lack of interest and investment in the client.

5. The client recumbent on a couch while talking with the counselor.
NOT USEFUL (-1)

This posture would not be effective for an intake session, unless a client personally requested it or was not feeling well.

RESPONSE DEVELOPMENT:

Using an appropriate pattern of questioning and an optimal spatial arrangement, the client now reveals his concerns. He has been driving a delivery truck for nearly one year. He now knows the route very well and is comfortable with his assignments. However, in recent months he has begun to experience problems. He has had a recurrent fantasy or "daydream" of what it would be like to "go back in time" with modern accouterments (his vehicle, clothing, knowledge, and the like). While the fantasy was just "good fun" in the beginning, it has begun to "take over" his thinking. Recently, it has become so intrusive and preoccupying that he has begun missing deliveries and is less than fully safe on the road. He is seeking help in coping with this situation. As he speaks, it is clear that he is embarrassed about what is happening, and yet overwhelmed by it enough to seek help. He is fearful of losing his job, or perhaps even getting in an accident and injuring others and himself.

Section C: Diagnostic Formulation.

Identify the most likely diagnosis, given the available information.

DIRECTIONS: Select the single most likely diagnosis in this situation. Check your answer. If your answer is not the one indicated write down your point value, then choose another answer and check your score again. Your score from this section will be the numbers added together. (For example: If your first choice was not indicated and had a score of -1, and your second answer choice was the one indicated with a score of +3, your score for this section would be a +2.)

- ☐ 1. Generalized Anxiety Disorder (F41.1)
- ☐ 2. Adjustment Disorder with Mixed Disturbance of Emotions and Conduct (F43.25).
- ☐ 3. Other psychoactive substance abuse with psychoactive substance-induced anxiety disorder (F19.180).
- ☐ 4. Acute Stress Reaction (F43.0).
- ☐ 5. Dissociative Identity Disorder (F44.81).
- ☐ 6. Obsessive-Compulsive Disorder, unspecified (F42.9).

NOW GO TO SECTION D.

Section C: Relevance of Diagnosis Options.

1. Generalized Anxiety Disorder (F41.1).
NOT INDICATED (-1)

The client's issue is very specific, and beyond this diagnostic category.

2. Adjustment Disorder with Mixed Disturbance of Emotions and Conduct (F43.25).
NOT INDICATED (-1)

If any other mental disorder better fits the symptoms, then this diagnosis must not be applied. In this situation, there is a better fit.

3. Other psychoactive substance abuse with psychoactive substance-induced anxiety disorder (F19.180).
NOT INDICATED (-2)

There is no indication of substance abuse.

4. Acute Stress Reaction (F43.0).
NOT INDICATED (-1)

There is no precipitating "traumatic event," which is the core feature of this diagnosis.

5. Dissociative Identity Disorder (F44.81).
NOT INDICATED (-1)

For this diagnosis, there is a discontinuity of the client's sense of self. There is no evidence of more than one personality state in this client.

6. Obsessive-Compulsive Disorder, unspecified (F42.9).
INDICATED (+3)

This client's issues properly fit the "obsessive" features of this disorder. His obsession involves: 1) recurrent and persistent thoughts, impulses, or images that are experienced, at some time during the disturbance, as intrusive and inappropriate and that cause marked anxiety or distress; 2) the thoughts, impulses, or images are not simply excessive worries about real-life problems; 3) the person attempts to ignore or suppress such thoughts, impulses, or images, or to neutralize them with some other thought or action. This client recognizes that the obsessional thoughts, impulses, or images are a product of his or her own mind, which would specify that this is with good or fair insight.

Section D: Optimum Treatment Modality.

From among the following, indicate the best treatment approach.

DIRECTIONS: Select the TWO most appropriate options provided in this Section. Check your answers. If your answers are not the ones indicated, write down your point value, then choose another answer and check your score again. Your score from this section will be the scores of all of your selections added together.

- □ 1. Engage the client in insight-oriented psychotherapy.
- □ 2. Provide cognitive-behavioral therapy.
- □ 3. Refer the client for electro-convulsive therapy.
- □ 4. Refer the client for a medications evaluation.
- □ 5. Begin a regimen of behavioral therapy.

NOW GO TO SECTION E.

Section D: Options Review and Findings:

1. Engage the client in insight-oriented psychotherapy.
NOT INDICATED (-3)

Insight-oriented psychotherapy has a poor track record in modifying OCD symptoms over the long term, although it may offer some short-term emotional benefits and support.

2. Provide cognitive-behavioral therapy.
INDICATED (+2)

Because the client's issue is primarily a thought-based obsession (as opposed to a behaviorally-based compulsion), this therapeutic approach is optimal. Using a cognitive restructuring approach, the client can be assisted in identifying the various triggers and disruptive thoughts associated with his obsession, and can learn to replace them with more realistic, functional thoughts. Given that the issues is being caught relatively early (involving only months, rather than years), the restructuring process should be relatively swift and very successful.

3. Refer the client for electro-convulsive therapy.
NOT INDICATED (-1)

This approach is sometimes used in cases of Obsessive-Compulsive Disorder, but it is not typically a first-choice approach. Other techniques and approaches are normally attempted first.

4. Refer the client for a medications evaluation.
INDICATED (+2)

The use of anti-depressant medication can be a particularly effective adjunct in the treatment of Obsessive-Compulsive Disorder. Therefore, a referral for a medications evaluation would be most appropriate. If prescribed, a monitoring and feedback component would be an important part of any treatment plan.

5. Begin a regimen of behavioral therapy.
NOT INDICATED (-2)

Behavioral therapy alone is more appropriate for situations where persistent compulsions are evident. However, where behavioral compulsions are absent, as in this scenario, the process of cognitive restructuring is a necessary addition to any behavioral treatment components used.

Section E: During the client's medication evaluation, you discover that the psychiatrist you normally refer to is unavailable, and another clinician is temporarily cross-covering her referrals. Upon returning, your client informs you that the cross-cover psychiatrist has enrolled him in a medications study to investigate the effectiveness of a new medication. He has been randomized into a group that could receive either a placebo or the investigational medication. Describe an appropriate first response to this information.

DIRECTIONS: Select the one most appropriate first response in this situation. Check your answer. If your answer is not the one indicated write down your point value, then choose another answer and check your score again. Your score from this section will be the numbers added together. (For example: If your first choice was not indicated and had a score of -1, and your second answer choice was the one indicated with a score of +3, your score for this section would be a +2.)

- ☐ 1. Rely on the investigational physician to resolve any subsequent concerns about Mark's treatment via the research study.
- ☐ 2. Ask Mark if he understands the purpose of the study.
- ☐ 3. Tell Mark that he needs to drop out of the study if he intends to continue working with you.
- ☐ 4. Consult with the physician (via information release) about Mark's safety concerns in driving.

Section E: Disposition Relevance and Rationale Formulation.

1. Rely on the investigational physician to resolve any subsequent concerns about Mark's treatment via the research study.

NOT INDICATED (-2)

It is not appropriate for a counselor to abdicate responsibility for a client's health and well-being simply because the client has been enrolled in a study. The ACA Code of Ethics Section G.1.f reminds counselors that although the "ultimate responsibility for ethical research lies with the principal researcher," it is essential that "others involved in the research activities" be "ethically... responsible for their own actions."

2. Ask Mark if he understands the purpose of the study.

NOT INDICATED (-1)

While some discussion of the client's understanding of the study may be in order, it is not the most pressing issue for further address. As emphasized in the ACA Code of Ethics Section A.2.b, requires that a counselor take reasonable "steps to ensure that clients understand the implications" of any intervention being used.

3. Tell Mark that he needs to drop out of the study if he intends to continue working with you.

NOT INDICATED (-1)

ACA Code of Ethics Section G introduction states that a counselor should "support the efforts of researchers by participating fully and willingly whenever possible." Undermining a research study without clear cause would not necessarily advance either the patient's best interests or the profession. This action could also undermine ACA Code of Ethics Section D.1.b., which states that counselors should "work to develop and strengthen relationships with colleagues from other disciplines to best serve clients."

4. Consult with the physician (via information release) about Mark's safety concerns in driving.

INDICATED (+3)

By enrolling the client in the investigational study, the possibility exists that the client will be randomized into a placebo (no medical treatment) group. This could result in the client receiving less than adequate available treatment. Given that the client has explicitly stated he fears for his driving safety when engaged in his obsessive thoughts, this concern must be addressed further. Specifically, the ACA Code of Ethics Section G.1.e. stipulates a counselor must "take reasonable precautions to avoid causing emotional, physical, or social harm to participants." The ACA Code of Ethics Section D, emphasizes the need for a formal information release for consultation between colleagues to take place.

SCORING: (Max = maximum possible; MPL = minimum passing level)

3A. Max 4; MPL 3
3B. Max 4; MPL 3
3C. Max 3; MPL 2
3D. Max 4; MPL 3
3E. Max 3; MPL 2

Simulation #4

A mother brings in her 15-year-old son, Steve, with complaints of frequent mood changes, belligerence, weight loss (12 lbs.), and a sharp drop-off in his performance in school. He was also dropped from the wrestling team, as he seemed to be having trouble keeping up during practice sessions, and was beginning to perform poorly at competitive events. On a few occasions, the mother noticed that Steve had signs of slurred speech and evidence of poor coordination, yet there was no odor of alcohol. Finally, he seems to be frequently mildly confused, and she doesn't know what to think of this.

NOW GO TO SECTION A.

Section A: Initial Information Gathering.

What intake information should be obtained and assessed to formulate a provisional diagnosis?

DIRECTIONS: Select as many as you consider indicated in this section. After making your selections and scoring your answers, it is beneficial to read the rationales and extended scenarios for all answer choices.

- ☐ 1. History of past athletic endeavors and achievements.
- ☐ 2. Past and current eating patterns and appetite.
- ☐ 3. Current behavioral problems.
- ☐ 4. Changes in hygiene and grooming.
- ☐ 5. Quality of social and family relationships.
- ☐ 6. Exploration of self-esteem issues.
- ☐ 7. Number and order of siblings in family of origin.
- ☐ 8. Health and medical history.
- ☐ 9. Current psychosocial stressors.
- ☐ 10. Changes in sleep patterns.

NOW GO TO SECTION B.

Section A: Element Relevance and Initial Information Obtained:

1. History of past athletic endeavors and achievements.
NOT INDICATED (-2)

Although the client has a history of participation in various athletic events (the mother indicates past participation in soccer, baseball, and swimming prior to wrestling), it is sufficient to know of this history and further details are not necessary.

2. Past and current eating patterns and appetite.
INDICATED (+1)

The client has lost about 12 lbs., according to the mother. "Making weight" often requires young wrestlers to lose weight in order to wrestle in their optimum weight class. This is often accomplished via heavy dieting, exercise, and occasional "purging" after eating to makeweight just prior to a competition "weighing-in" event. This client, however, denies dieting, major exercise, and purging to make weight before or after being discharged from the team. When asked why he's lost weight, the client responds only, "I don't know."

3. Current behavioral problems.
INDICATED (+2)

The client will not admit to or discuss any behavioral issues. However, his mother notes that he has been behaving erratically for about the last six months. Behavior problems have included: failing to return home after school, insisting on staying out at friends' homes, leaving the home without permission late at night, refusing to complete homework assignments, avoiding family contact (particularly the mother), refusing chores, and belligerently refusing to talk. The mother also voiced concerns about the "friends he's running with." She noted specifically, "I think he's involved in some sort of pre-gang-like 'graffiti' activity. I keep finding spray paint cans hidden in his room, and even in his school pack. They call it 'tagging,' and he says he'll never get caught, but I keep taking the cans away from him anyway."

4. Changes in hygiene and grooming.
INDICATED (+1)

The client presents as clean and well groomed, and the mother indicates that he has always been particular about his appearance. Apparently, this has not changed.

5. Quality of social and family relationships.
INDICATED (+1)

The client has been avoiding all family members (he has three younger siblings), and home life in general. His parents divorced when he was about nine years of age, and the father has largely remained absent over the ensuing six years. No new contact or conflicts with the father were noted. The client's belligerence and refusal to talk with the mother is relatively new. Prior to the last six months, he was generally approachable, particularly prior to starting high school. In terms of social relationships, the mother has noted that the client's circle of friends seems to have diminished markedly. While he had many friends in the past, it now seems that he's only maintaining relationships with two key friends, and the others have fallen out of contact.

6. Exploration of self-esteem issues.
NOT INDICATED (-2)

Although the client has experienced recent losses (discharge from the wrestling team, failing grades, and a narrowing circle of friends), self-esteem issues are not likely to be at the root of the client's current presentation.

7. Number and order of siblings in family of origin.
NOT INDICATED (-2)

The birth order and number of siblings is unlikely to have any bearing on the presenting problem.

8. Health and medical history.
INDICATED (+2)

Very relevant. There is nothing, however, in the client's health and medical history to clarify the current changes. All developmental markers were normal to this point in his life, he has had only typical childhood diseases, and the physical examination he obtained eight months prior, for clearance to join the wrestling team, was unremarkable.

9. Current psychosocial stressors.
NOT INDICATED (-1)

There is no indication that there are any unusual psychosocial stressors that would be disrupting the client's life.

10. Changes in sleep patterns.
NOT INDICATED (-1)

There is no indication that the client is experiencing any particular sleep problem.

FORMULATION AND INITIAL FOLLOW-UP: The client's intake clinical picture is challenging due to overall non-responsiveness. Concerns include: 1) physical compromise (reports of poor stamina and loss of his competitive edge); 2) unexplained weight loss; 3) mood changes; 4) episodes of slurred speech and decreased motor coordination not explained by alcohol use; and 5) mild confusion. All these factors strongly indicate the need for a medical evaluation. Other concerning signs: 1) belligerence; 2) loss of most friends; 3) non-alcohol-based slurred speech and ataxia; and 4) the frequent presence of aerosol paint cans; and 5) protracted intake-response pattern to questions.

This page is intentionally blank.

Section B: Based on the intake data, Identify the most likely diagnosis, given the available information.

DIRECTIONS: Select the single most likely diagnosis in this situation. Check your answer. If your answer is not the one indicated write down your point value, then choose another answer and check your score again. Your score from this section will be the numbers added together. (For example: If your first choice was not indicated and had a score of -1, and your second answer choice was the one indicated with a score of +3, your score for this section would be a +2.)

- ☐ 1. Schizophrenia, unspecified (F20.9).
- ☐ 2. Conduct Disorder, Adolescent-Onset Type (F91.2).
- ☐ 3. Oppositional Defiant Disorder (F91.3).
- ☐ 4. Adjustment Disorder with Mixed Disturbance of Emotions and Conduct (F43.25).
- ☐ 5. Conduct Disorder, unspecified (F91.9).
- ☐ 6. Illness, unspecified (R69).

NOW GO TO SECTION C.

Section B: Based upon the intake information available, identify a tentative intake diagnostic impression:

1. Schizophrenia, unspecified. (F20.9).
NOT INDICATED (-1)

There is no evidence of attention to internal stimuli, and hygiene and grooming are good (which tends to rule out psychosis). The client is also fairly young for a schizophrenic break, with age at onset typically around 18 for males and 25 for females.

2. Conduct Disorder, Adolescent-Onset Type (F91.2).
NOT INDICATED (-1)

Behavior does not include violence, aggression, use of weapons, etc.; no clear evidence of destruction of property (graffiti is an assumption, and does not include outright destruction and/or fire setting); does stay out at night, but this behavior did not begin before age 13; does not run away from home, and school truancy has not been reported.

3. Oppositional Defiant Disorder (F91.3).
NOT INDICATED (-1)

Symptoms have not yet persisted longer than six months, and the potential for a mood disorder, substance use, or a psychotic disorder has not yet been ruled out.

4. Adjustment Disorder with Mixed Disturbance of Emotions and Conduct (F43.25).
NOT INDICATED (-1)

There is no identifiable "stressor" to which an adjustment is being required.

5. Conduct Disorder, unspecified (F91.9).
NOT INDICATED (-1)

This diagnostic category is typically used when criteria for both Conduct Disorder and Oppositional Defiant Disorder are present, but where the behavioral symptoms have not reached threshold criteria for either. This adolescent, however, seems to lack the violence, aggression, destructive behaviors, vengeful goals, and other criteria that would warrant this diagnostic label.

6. Illness, unspecified (R69).
INDICATED (+3)

Given the many questions remaining, it would appear most appropriate to defer a diagnosis.

Section C: Additional Information Gathering.

What additional information should be obtained and assessed to formulate a provisional diagnosis?

DIRECTIONS: Select as many as you consider indicated in this section. After making your selections and scoring your answers, it is beneficial to read the rationales and extended scenarios for all answer choices.

- ☐ 1. In-depth coach report.
- ☐ 2. In-depth teacher report.
- ☐ 3. Urine and blood drug testing
- ☐ 4. Medical evaluation and report.
- ☐ 5. Sibling interviews.
- ☐ 6. Legal history review.

NOW GO TO SECTION D.

Section C: Element Relevance and Additional Information Obtained.

1. In-depth coach report.
INDICATED (+1)

Upon further questioning the coach specified that the client seemed to either be malingering or else he "wasn't feeling himself." He indicated that the client was lethargic, apathetic, and seemed unable to "react quick enough" to compete effectively. Further, he seemed to have trouble remembering and following instructions.

2. In-depth teacher report.
INDICATED (+1)

Several of the client's teachers were questioned, and each expressed concern over the client's declining performance and grades. Each noted that the client was having difficulty concentrating, attending to assigned tasks, and following instructions. One teacher was sufficiently concerned to have made a referral to the school psychologist, but the evaluation was still pending.

3. Urine and blood drug testing.
NOT INDICATED (-1)

The client denies the use of any "street drugs." No information indicates otherwise, and therefore, laboratory testing for drugs would not normally be pursued at this early juncture.

4. Medical evaluation and report.
INDICATED (+2)

The client has unexplained weight loss, decreased stamina (per discharge from the wrestling team), episodes of unexplained slurred speech and poor coordination, and some evidence of mild confusion. Further evaluation is difficult, as the client offers one- and two-word answers to questions, and he refuses to participate in any further evaluation at the time of intake. Some irregular pauses were noted between questions asked and client responses, but it is difficult to determine what may be causing this. A medical evaluation is certainly indicated.

5. Siblings interview.
INDICATED (+1)

Collateral contact with the client's siblings offers additional insights. The next closest child in age, a 14-year-old brother, cites friends who state the client has been "hanging out with glue-heads." Asked what that means, he clarifies the reference as being youths who "sniff stuff to get high." In further inquiry, both the sibling and his mother note not only aerosol cans among the client's things, but an unusual number of "white-out" bottles, tubes and bottles of glue, and other products containing volatile vaporous solvents and compounds.

6. Legal history review.
NOT INDICATED (-2)

There is no indication of legal problems.

RESPONSE DEVELOPMENT:

Given the additional information, there is a primary concern of inhalant abuse: "sniffing" (direct inhalation from a container), "huffing" (inhalation from a substance-soaked rag), and/or "bagging" (inhalation of a substance placed in a paper or plastic bag). Inquiring further, the mother notes an "odd chemical smell" was often evident on the client's breath and person. When confronted with this information, the client admitted to frequent inhalant use involving multiple substances. The mother reported this during further medical evaluation by both the client's pediatrician and a neurologist. The findings: potentially permanent neurological damage secondary to inhalant abuse, and brain damage due to episodes of hypoxia (lack of oxygen) and acute and cumulative solvent toxicity. Impairments included decreased executive functioning (e.g., problems with abstracting, planning, organizing, and sequencing information and events), aphasia (language disturbance), apraxia (impaired coordination and movement), and impaired memory and learning capacity.

This page is intentionally blank.

Section D: Provisional Diagnosis Formulation.

Based upon the available information, what would appear to be the most appropriate primary provisional diagnosis?

DIRECTIONS: Select the most appropriate primary diagnosis indicated in this section. Check your answer. If your answer is not the one indicated write down your point value, then choose another answer and check your score again. Your score from this section will be the numbers added together. (For example: If your first choice was not indicated and had a score of -1, and your second answer choice was the one indicated with a score of +3, your score for this section would be a +2.)

- ☐ 1. Mild Cognitive Impairment (G31.84).
- ☐ 2. Unspecified Intellectual Disability (F79).
- ☐ 3. Specific Developmental Disorder of Motor Function (F82).
- ☐ 4. Inhalant Use, unspecified (F18.90).
- ☐ 5. Illness, unspecified (R69).
- ☐ 6. Inhalant use, unspecified with Inhalant-Induced Psychotic Disorder, unspecified (F18.959).

NOW GO TO SECTION E.

Section D: Relevance and Diagnostic Formulation.

1. Mild Cognitive Impairment (G31.84).
NOT INDICATED (-1)

Although this client has experienced a significant decline in cognitive functioning, this is not the primary focus of clinical attention.

2. Unspecified Intellectual Disability (F79).
NOT INDICATED (-1)

The DSM indicates that, diagnostically, intellectual disability may emerge "from whatever cause." However, it is invariably related to developmental factors that occur before the age of 18. Although this client is under the age of 18, the precipitating cause of his cognitive change is not "developmental" in nature (i.e., occurring from factors relevant to the maturational process). Further, no information about the client's Intelligence Quotient (IQ) threshold is available, and there is not sufficient evidence of adaptive functioning deficits in the client at this time.

3. Specific Developmental Disorder of Motor Function (F82).
NOT INDICATED (-1)

Numerous individuals have noted episodes of poor motor coordination in the client's presentation at various times. However, it is not clear how pronounced the condition is when the client is not impaired due to inhalant use, nor is the condition "developmental" in nature.

4. Inhalant Use, unspecified (F18.90).
INDICATED (+3)

This is the condition of clinical focus, and the client meets all criteria necessary for the application of this diagnosis.

5. Illness, unspecified (R69).
NOT INDICATED (-1)

The client does exhibit specific features of behavior that warrant a diagnosis.

6. Inhalant use, unspecified with Inhalant-Induced Psychotic Disorder, unspecified (F18.959).
NOT INDICATED (-1)

While the client may well have experienced episodes of psychosis when using inhalants, there was no evidence of psychosis during any evaluative period. Therefore, this would not be the primary diagnosis. Should the client reveal past psychotic episodes, it would still not be the primary diagnosis, but could be logged as a "by history" diagnostic entry.

Section E: Decision Making.

Identify the services you can provide to help the client.

DIRECTIONS: Select the most appropriate options provided in this section. After making your selections and scoring your answers, it is beneficial to read the rationales and extended scenarios for all answer choices.

- □ 1. Referral to a 12-step addiction recovery program.
- □ 2. Psychiatric hospitalization.
- □ 3. Support group referral for the client and family.
- □ 4. Neuropsychological testing for learning and cognition.
- □ 5. A two-day detoxification program.
- □ 6. Individual counseling to cope with related issues.

Section E: Options Relevance and Findings.

1. Referral to a 12-step addiction recovery program.
INDICATED (+1)

Standard substance abuse treatment programs will be unable to address the multiple problems that accompany inhalant abuse. Not only is chronic inhalant abuse accompanied by numerous psychological and social problems, but the sequelae of neurological damage often results in a dual diagnosis of chemical dependency and mental illness, with unique limits in learning and capacity for change. Therefore, referral to a program specific to inhalant abuse is strongly recommended.

2. Psychiatric hospitalization.
NOT INDICATED (-1)

Inhalant abuse can lead to both psychological and physiological dependence and withdrawal problems, but there is no report of this client experiencing these problems. Thus, hospitalization would not be indicated. Further, the client's abuse history appears to be only months in duration, making hospitalization concerns less acute.

3. Support group referral for the client and family.
INDICATED (+2)

Both the client and his family could benefit from a support group referral, both to assist in learning about the condition and it treatment, and for additional psychological and social support during the treatment process.

4. Neuropsychological testing for learning and cognition.
INDICATED (+1)

Neurological problems are common in situations of inhalant abuse. Both early and later testing can be important, to follow changes in capacity over time. Inhalant toxins accumulate in the fatty tissues of the body, and recovery and healing can occur over a considerable duration of time. Therefore, repeat testing to optimize the treatment intervention process is essential.

5. A two-day detoxification program.
NOT INDICATED (-1)

No issues of physiological dependence or withdrawal have been identified in this client. However, where such issues do emerge, detoxification of inhalants will require much more than 2-3 day period. Inhalant toxins accumulate in the fatty tissues of the body and will continue to be released for many weeks. Thus, more protracted detoxification is necessary, if it is to be effective.

6. Individual counseling to cope with related issues.
INDICATED (+2)

Most clients abusing inhalants have numerous underlying personal, familial, and/or social problems that need to be addressed. Without work on these collateral issues of concern, the client is very likely to relapse shortly after release.

SCORING: (Max = maximum possible; MPL = minimum passing level)

4A. Max 7; MPL 5
4B. Max 3; MPL 2
4C. Max 5; MPL 4
4D. Max 3; MPL 2
4E. Max 6; MPL 5

This page is intentionally blank.

Simulation #5

You are in private practice, and a mother brings in her 17-year-old daughter, Ellen. The presenting complaint is that the daughter has been accusing virtually everyone in the home of "talking about her behind her back." Any verbal exchange leads the daughter to believe that some secret, pejorative dialogue about her is occurring. Further, other emotive episodes (laughter, arguing, anger, etc.) are all interpreted by the daughter as being about her, when they are not. The problem has escalated over the past 2-3 weeks, and recently spilled over into the school environment, with the daughter accusing classmates, teachers, and others of similar behavior. Most recently she has been seen and heard talking to herself, sometimes in a highly animated fashion. Upon meeting you, she smiles oddly and then declares that she knows "exactly what you're thinking." When you inquire further, her expression changes to one of intense distrust and anger, and she refuses to disclose her feelings further.

NOW GO TO SECTION A.

Section A: Initial Information Gathering.

What initial information would be most important in formulating a provisional DSM diagnosis?

DIRECTIONS: Select as many as you consider indicated. After making your selections and scoring your answers, it is beneficial to read the rationales and extended scenarios for all answer choices.

- ☐ 1. Intelligence quotient testing.
- ☐ 2. An evaluation of past eating patterns and weight changes.
- ☐ 3. Past psychiatric history.
- ☐ 4. Academic performance history.
- ☐ 5. Childhood illnesses.
- ☐ 6. Historical changes in mood and emotions.
- ☐ 7. Roster of current hobbies.
- ☐ 8. Past and current substance abuse history.

NOW GO TO SECTION B.

Section A: Element Relevance and Initial Information Obtained.

1. Intelligence quotient testing.
NOT INDICATED (-3)

There is no indication of cognitive impairment.

2. An evaluation of past eating patterns and weight changes.
NOT INDICATED (-2)

There is no indication that the client's weight has fluctuated, nor that she has any form of eating problem.

3. Psychiatric history.
INDICATED (+2)

The client is not currently responding to questions, but the mother is able to clarify that the client has no prior psychiatric history. Typically, the daughter is responsive, responsible, thoughtful, and even-tempered. Consequently, this behavior is highly irregular and well outside the client's normal repertoire of conduct.

4. Academic performance history.
INDICATED (+2)

The client has an outstanding academic performance record. She invariably makes excellent grades, and is often the recipient of praise from her teachers and others.

5. Childhood illnesses.
NOT INDICATED (-2)

There is nothing to suggest that any childhood illnesses are related to the client's presentation in way.

6. Historical changes in mood and emotions.
NOT INDICATED (-1)

The mother indicates that the client has always been even-tempered, calm, pleasant, and positive. They have never had any problem with her being overly moody, dramatic, grandiose, or depressed.

7. Roster of current hobbies.
NOT INDICATED (-2)

There is no indication that the client's hobbies would be relevant to her current presentation.

8. Past and current substance abuse history.
INDICATED (+2)

The mother reports that the daughter has never used illicit drugs in the past, nor has she associated with friends who have used drugs. Further, the client is not taking any prescription or over-the-counter medications of any kind.

RESPONSE DEVELOPMENT:

This client presents as historically very stable and with a high level of personal performance and excellent academic and social functioning. There is no history of past psychiatric problems, and no history of substance abuse. Very recently the client underwent a substantial change in mood, affect, and behavior. Her mood became very suspicious, paranoid, and secretive. Her affect has reportedly been very labile and often incongruent with her mood and verbal expressions. Her behavior has been indicative of agitation, distrust, attention to internal stimuli, and self-isolation.

This page is intentionally blank.

Section B: Based upon the intake data, identify potential diagnoses needing further exploration.

DIRECTIONS: Select as many as seem appropriate at this evaluative juncture. After making your selections and scoring your answers, it is beneficial to read the rationales and extended scenarios for all answer choices.

- ☐ 1. Brief Psychotic Disorder (F23).
- ☐ 2. Cyclothymic Disorder (F34.0).
- ☐ 3. Other Psychoactive Substance Use, unspecified with unspecified Psychoactive Substance-Induced Disorder (F19.99).
- ☐ 4. Bipolar Disorder, Current Episode Manic Severe with Psychotic Features (F31.2).
- ☐ 5. Schizophreniform Disorder (F20.81).
- ☐ 6. Intermittent Explosive Disorder (F63.81).
- ☐ 7. Schizophrenia, unspecified (F20.9).
- ☐ 8. Major Depressive Disorder, Single Episode, Severe with Psychotic Features (F32.3).

NOW GO TO SECTION C.

Section B: Diagnostic Relevance and Further Information.

1. Brief psychotic disorder (F23).
INDICATED (+2)

By all appearances and reports the client is attending to internal stimuli ("voices," and/or grappling with other delusions, hallucinations, etc.). The duration of the problem is currently less than one month, and it is not in response to any apparent precipitating stressors.

2. Cyclothymic disorder (F34.0).
NOT INDICATED (-2)

This diagnosis requires evidence of both hypomanic and depressive symptoms (short of major depression) for a period of two years. Certainly this client's symptoms are both very new in onset and very severe. Therefore, this would not be a potential diagnosis.

3. Other Psychoactive Substance Use, unspecified with unspecified Psychoactive Substance-Induced Disorder (F19.99).
NOT INDICATED (-1)

There is no indication of substance abuse. The possibility cannot be ruled out entirely, but the information provided offers no such indication.

4. Bipolar Disorder, Current Episode Manic Severe with Psychotic Features (F31.2).
INDICATED (+1)

It is possible that the client is experiencing a manic episode severe enough to precipitate psychotic features. Even so, this diagnosis would appear less likely, given her pre-morbid level of function and the absence of any prior psychiatric history.

5. Schizophreniform Disorder (F20.81).
INDICATED (+1)

This diagnosis remains a possibility. The diagnosis requires that parts A, D, and E of Schizophrenia must be met. The client meets criteria for part "A" of schizophrenia, as the client apparently hears "voices" virtually continuously in her mind and also presents with negative symptoms. Part "D" remains to be seen, as some mood incongruencies exist, but are as of yet very brief and therefore, may not be determinative. Part "E" also appears to be met, as there is no link to medications or substance abuse. However, the condition must also resolve within a period of six months or less, and this is yet to be determined. The potential is good, however, given the fact that the client's pre-morbid level of functioning is very good and there is no psychiatric history.

6. Intermittent Explosive Disorder (F63.81).
NOT INDICATED (-2)

There is no indication that there have been any "serious assaultive acts or destruction of property." Consequently, it would not appear that this diagnosis will remain relevant.

7. Schizophrenia, unspecified (F20.9).
INDICATED (+2)

Early indications suggest that the client may well meet criteria for schizophrenia. The Criteria for part "A" appear to be met, given the client's apparent attention to some form of "voices" that seem to constantly keep up a running dialogue in the client's mind. Part B criteria are also met, as social and academic functioning appear to be deleteriously affected. Part C, however, is lacking, as the duration is currently very brief (i.e., less than the requisite 6 months).

8. Major Depressive Disorder, Single Episode, Severe With Psychotic Features (F32.3).
NOT INDICATED (-1)

While the client does exhibit some moodiness, it does not appear to be primarily depressive in nature. Therefore, in spite of the presence of apparent psychotic symptoms, this diagnosis is unlikely to be related or sustained.

This page is intentionally blank.

Section C: Additional Information Gathering.

What next steps might be indicated for this client?

DIRECTIONS: Select as many as you consider indicated in this section. After making your selections and scoring your answers, it is beneficial to read the rationales and extended scenarios for all answer choices.

- ☐ 1. Referral for a medical evaluation.
- ☐ 2. The Mental Status Exam (MSE).
- ☐ 3. Referral for a medications evaluation.
- ☐ 4. Rorschach Psychodiagnostic Testing.
- ☐ 5. Psychiatric hospitalization.
- ☐ 6. Beck Depression Inventory-II (BDI-II).

NOW GO TO SECTION D.

Section C: Relevance of Proposed Assessment Tools and Interventions.

1. Referral for a medical evaluation.
INDICATED (+2)

Medical evaluation in situations of this nature is always indicated. It is necessary to ensure that there are no metabolic, endocrinological, electrolyte, thyroid, or other disorders that might precipitate the symptoms. In this case, all laboratory findings and drug screens were negative, there was no evidence of trauma, and the physical exam was also unremarkable.

2. The Mental Status Exam (MSE).
INDICATED (+2)

The Mental Status Exam is designed to reveal evidence of cognitive deficits in attention, concentration, and memory; impairments in executive functioning, insight and judgment; abnormalities in consciousness, orientation, speech, mood, and affect; as well as addressing suicidality, homicidality, and psychotic features such as hallucinations, delusions, and other perceptual and cognitive distortions. While the client was not fully cooperative with the exam, she did reveal that she was hearing voices that suggested others were speaking badly of her. Although distressed at this, she denied any desire toward self-harm or harming others.

3. Referral for a medications evaluation.
INDICATED (+2)

Psychotic symptoms can be very distressing, and medications can be immensely helpful in slowing down racing thoughts, reducing auditory hallucinations and concurrent agitation, and generally imposing a greater feeling of security and calm. Therefore, a referral to a psychiatrist for a medications evaluation is of paramount importance.

4. Rorschach Psychodiagnostic Testing.
NOT INDICATED (-2)

This projective assessment tool is used in uncovering useful unconscious material. However, its administration requires that an individual be cognitively intact and free of psychotic symptomatology in order to respond to the ink-blot images. Given this client's situation, Rorschach testing would not be productive.

5. Psychiatric hospitalization.
NOT INDICATED (-1)

The client denies "command" auditory hallucinations, suicidality, and homicidality. She also remains at home under the supervision of family. The medications evaluation is in progress. Thus, there appears to be no imminent need of psychiatric hospitalization.

6. Beck Depression Inventory-II (BDI-II).
NOT INDICATED (-1)

There is no indication that the client is primarily depressed.

FORMULATION: Four months pass and the client makes gradual but steady improvement. Psychotropic medications have been in place during this time, and appear to be effective. At five months, the client begins to be titrated off her medications, and there appears to be no recurrence of the auditory hallucinations. By six months, she is back to her usual high-functioning baseline.

This page is intentionally blank.

Section D: Based on the information above, what final diagnosis would be appropriate for this client?

DIRECTIONS: Select the one most appropriate primary diagnosis. Check your answer. If your answer is not the one indicated write down your point value, then choose another answer and check your score again. Your score from this section will be the numbers added together. (For example: If your first choice was not indicated and had a score of -1, and your second answer choice was the one indicated with a score of +3, your score for this section would be a +2.)

- ☐ 1. Generalized Anxiety Disorder (F41.1).
- ☐ 2. Acute Stress Reaction (F43.0).
- ☐ 3. Bipolar Disorder, Current Episode Manic Severe with Psychotic Features (F31.2).
- ☐ 4. Schizophreniform Disorder (F20.81).
- ☐ 5. Schizophrenia, unspecified (F20.9).
- ☐ 6. Brief psychotic disorder (F23).

Section D: Element Relevance and Diagnostic Formulation.

1. Generalized Anxiety Disorder (F41.1).
NOT INDICATED (-2)

The client is not experiencing excessive anxiety and worry about "a number of events or activities," nor has the condition exceeded "at least 6 months" duration. Therefore, this would not be an appropriate diagnosis.

2. Acute Stress Reaction (F43.0).
NOT INDICATED (-1)

The client has not experienced a traumatic event or events that involved a threat of death or serious injury to herself or others. Therefore, this would not be an appropriate diagnosis.

3. Bipolar Disorder, Current Episode Manic Severe With Psychotic Features (F31.2).
NOT INDICATED (-1)

The client had some early evidence of moodiness early on, but it lacked the extreme depressive and/or grandiosity characteristic of a bipolar episode. Therefore, in spite of the presence of psychotic features, this would not be the appropriate diagnosis.

4. Schizophreniform Disorder (F20.81).
INDICATED (+3)

The client met criteria A, D, and E for schizophrenia (A: auditory hallucinations; D: mood disorders were ruled out, due to an absence of symptoms; and E: substance abuse and medical conditions were also ruled out). Finally, the condition lasted for longer than a month and yet less than six months. The specifier "with good prognostic features" applies because: a) the client's symptoms became acute in less than four weeks, and b) the client had excellent premorbid academic and social functioning.

5. Schizophrenia, unspecified (F20.9).
NOT INDICATED (-1)

Although the client exhibited many of the features characteristic of schizophrenia, including some measure of paranoia, the condition did not meet criterion C — "continuous signs of the disturbance persist for at least 6 months." Therefore, this would not be the proper diagnosis.

6. Brief psychotic disorder (F23).
NOT INDICATED (-1)

The client met all criteria for this diagnosis except one – the condition did not resolve within one month or less. Therefore, this would not be an accurate diagnosis.

SCORING: (Max = maximum possible; MPL = minimum passing level)

5A. Max 6; MPL 4
5B. Max 6; MPL 4
5C. Max 6; MPL 4
5D. Max 3; MPL 2

Simulation #6

A 56 year old daughter brings in her 80-year-old mother, Marjorie, with a chief complaint of "cluttering and hoarding" to the point of dysfunction. The problem was brought to a head when the mother recently fell in the home and injured her knee. After a brief hospital visit, rehabilitative physical therapy was ordered, and a physical therapist was sent to the home, in company with the daughter, to prepare for the patient's discharge. To their dismay, the home was filled, virtually floor to ceiling with an amazing array of "stuff"—boxes of magazines, bins of clothing, piles of old newspapers, a variety of household items, cooking paraphernalia, health items, etc., still in their original unopened boxes; file cabinets filled with mail, advertisements, clippings, photocopies, bills, and other paperwork of a great variety; etc. The clutter extended throughout the home, and was significant enough that none of the three bedrooms could be entered, the bathroom was barely accessible (the bathtub was filled with things), the kitchen was unusable, and the living room had no negotiable space beyond that immediately around a recliner (in which the client clearly slept) and a television surrounded by boxes of second-hand video cassettes and some DVD movies. In the backyard were five metal sheds, all full, which had been erected by a son who had hoped each time to off-load some things and help the client become more functional. The daughter took her mother home during the rehabilitative period, but now is uncertain what to do to ensure her mother's safety.

NOW GO TO SECTION A.

Section A: Initial Information Gathering.

From among the following, identify those early questions that would be most appropriate to elicit the client's understanding of the presenting problem.

DIRECTIONS: Select as many as you consider correct. After making your selections and scoring your answers, it is beneficial to read the rationales and extended scenarios for all answer choices.

- ☐ 1. Do you know why you've been brought to see me today?
- ☐ 2. What's keeping you from cleaning up your house?
- ☐ 3. Can you tell me about your greatest concern today?
- ☐ 4. How do you feel about the physical therapy you received?
- ☐ 5. Do you know why others are concerned about your home situation?
- ☐ 6. Did you know that city fire hazard ordinances limit what you can store in your home?
- ☐ 7. Do you want me to call the authorities and report you?
- ☐ 8. What do you see as your options in your current situation?

NOW GO TO SECTION B.

Section A: Selection Relevance and Initial Information Obtained.

1. Do you know why you've been brought to see me today?
INDICATED (+2)

This question allows the client to express her own understanding of the visit. The client responded, "Yes, my children won't let me go back home, and you're here to help them keep me out."

2. What's keeping you from cleaning up your house?
NOT INDICATED (-2)

This is an abrupt, confrontational question that could easily generate antagonism between the client and the counselor.

3. Can you tell me about your greatest concern today?
INDICATED (+2)

This is a helpful question that gives the client ample opportunity to express her fears and concerns. The client responded, "My greatest concern is that I won't be allowed my personal freedom to live the way I want."

4. How do you feel about the physical therapy you received?
NOT INDICATED (-2)

This question simply evades the real issue.

5. Do you know why others are concerned about your home situation?
INDICATED (+3)

This is an important open-ended question. It allows the client to demonstrate her understanding of the views and concerns of others. The client responded, "They think I can't take care of myself. Well, I've been living alone since my husband died 12 years ago, and I think I do just fine."

6. Did you know that city fire hazard ordinances limit what you can store in your home?
INDICATED (+1)

Care needs to be used in asking this question, as it could easily be perceived as a threat. If asked thoughtfully, however, it can be a useful way of learning whether or not the client understands the significance of her situation. The client responded, "No, no one ever told me about this."

7. Do you want me to call the authorities and report you?
NOT INDICATED (-3)

This is a highly confrontational question, and poses a clear and immediate threat to the dialogue process.

8. What do you see as your options in your current situation?
INDICATED (+2)

This is a particularly useful open-ended question. It allows the client to begin the personal problem-solving process. The client responded, "I don't feel like I have any options."

Section B: Identify additional information needed to explore the client's capacity for insight into her current situation.

DIRECTIONS: Select all additional information likely to be helpful in exploring the client's capacity for insight into her current situation. After making your selections and scoring your answers, it is beneficial to read the rationales and extended scenarios for all answer choices.

- □ 1. Ask client: "What do you feel you need to do about things at home?"
- □ 2. Ask adult children: "Will your mother allow you to help her?"
- □ 3. Ask client: "What kinds of employment have you held in the past?"
- □ 4. Ask adult children: "Was your mother abusive as you grew up?"
- □ 5. Ask client: "Is there anything you feel you could donate or discard?"
- □ 6. Ask client: "Are you concerned about your safety and well-being in the home?"
- □ 7. Ask adult children: "In most things, is your mother rigid and inflexible, or open and accommodating?"
- □ 8. Ask client: "Do you feel your health is good, fair, or just poor?"
- □ 9. Ask adult children: "Would you describe your mother as highly focused on order, tasks, lists, and details?"
- □ 10. Ask adult children: "Is your mother what you might call a perfectionist, even in leisure or recreational activities?"

NOW GO TO SECTION C.

Section B: Relevance of additional information.

1. Ask client: "What do you feel you need to do about things at home?"
INDICATED (+2)

The client responded: "I don't think I need to do anything. Things are fine just as they are."

2. Ask adult children: "Will your mother allow you to help her?"
INDICATED (+1)

Both of her adult children noted, "No. She's always concerned that we'll do something wrong, throw something away, or mix up the 'order' of things in the house. It doesn't seem like there's any order to anything in the house, but she assures us there is and that we might somehow mess things up. Mom's always been this way. She's always been very particular about how things are done."

3. Ask client: "What kinds of employment have you held in the past?"
NOT INDICATED (-1)

There is no reason to believe this question will yield any particularly relevant information. In point of fact, she was a bookkeeper, and was very successful in that line of employment, given her eye for details.

4. Ask adult children: "Was your mother abusive as you grew up?"
NOT INDICATED (-2)

In terms of the issue being addressed, this is not a relevant question.

5. Ask client: "Is there anything you feel you could donate or discard?"
INDICATED (+2)

The client responded, "No. I only keep things that I want, and that I feel I can use or may someday need."

6. Ask client: "Are you concerned about your safety and well-being in the home?"
INDICATED (+2)

The client responded, "No more than anyone else in town. My home is just as safe as anyone else's."

7. Ask adult children: "In most things, is your mother rigid and inflexible, or open and accommodating?"
INDICATED (+1)

The adult children responded, "Mom's always been very loving and caring. She's a very sensitive and kind person, and has a good heart. However, there's no question that she's really rigid. There were lots of rules as we grew up, and she had no tolerance for any deviation from what she expected."

8. Ask client: "Do you feel your health is good, fair, or just poor?"
NOT INDICATED (-1)

This is not a particularly relevant question, given the issue being addressed.

9. Ask adult children: "Would you describe your mother as highly focused on order, tasks, lists, and details?"
INDICATED (+1)

The adult children responded, "Yes. She's always made highly detailed lists for everything. Also, everything has a very strict order, both in terms of how tasks and chores were done, and in terms of how things were put away in the home as we grew up. She didn't collect things then, like she does now. But we also couldn't afford much when we were growing up. It's just been since we left home that she started collecting things."

10. Ask adult children: "Is your mother what you might call a perfectionist, even in leisure or recreational activities?"
INDICATED (+1)

The adult children responded, "Mother's very much a perfectionist. She always worked hard to keep things just so. When it came to leisure or recreational time, Mom never really took a break. She was always busy, keeping things in order, cleaned, and ready to be used. If it wasn't for Dad, who liked taking vacations, I don't think she'd have ever left the house for much of anything—except occasional trips to see her own parents about every 5-6 years."

This page is intentionally blank.

Section C: Diagnostic Formulation.

Using solely the above information, identify the client's most likely diagnosis.

DIRECTIONS: Select the single most likely diagnosis in this situation. Check your answer. If your answer is not the one indicated write down your point value, then choose another answer and check your score again. Your score from this section will be the numbers added together. (For example: If your first choice was not indicated and had a score of -1, and your second answer choice was the one indicated with a score of +3, your score for this section would be a +2.)

- ☐ 1. Adjustment Disorder, With Depressed Mood (F43.21).
- ☐ 2. Hoarding Disorder (F42.3).
- ☐ 3. Adjustment Disorder, With Disturbance of Conduct (F43.24).
- ☐ 4. Generalized Anxiety Disorder (F41.1).
- ☐ 5. Obsessive-Compulsive Personality Disorder (F60.5).
- ☐ 6. Conduct Disorder, unspecified (F91.9).

NOW GO TO SECTION D.

Section C: Relevance of DSM diagnosis selected.

1. Adjustment Disorder, With Depressed Mood (F43.21).
NOT INDICATED (-2)

As there is no specific precipitating situation requiring "adjustment," and clear features of a mood disorder are absent, this would not be the proper diagnosis.

2. Hoarding Disorder (F42.3).
INDICATED (+3)

Hoarding Disorder was previously considered a symptom of OCD. However, now it is its own diagnosis. Hoarders have an obsession to acquire things they believe they will need and/or to keep valueless things they wonder if they "might" someday need, and/or to sort and organize repetitively, but without ever achieving order or discarding or putting away anything. This disorder can be classified as with good insight, poor insight, or absent insight.

3. Adjustment Disorder, With Disturbance of Conduct (F43.24).
NOT INDICATED (-2)

There is no specific precipitating situation requiring "adjustment," and the current behavioral features are certainly not associated with such a specific event. Therefore, this would not be an accurate diagnosis.

4. Generalized Anxiety Disorder (F41.1).
NOT INDICATED (-1)

This diagnosis is characterized by "excessive anxiety and worry" about multiple events, activities, or performance for a period in excess of six months. Further, the distress itself must have compromised social, occupational, or other important areas of functioning. Although the client is now voicing anxiety and worry, it is related solely to recent concerns about her home organization and the possible loss of her belongings. Therefore, her distress is not "generalized" to numerous events, activities or performance, nor has the distress persisted for longer than six months. Thus, this would not be the appropriate diagnosis.

5. Obsessive-Compulsive Personality Disorder (F60.5).
NOT INDICATED (-1)

The client clearly has "traits" of Obsessive-Compulsive Personality Disorder, particularly given the historical information supplied by her adult children. However, it is generally seen as poor clinical practice to diagnosis a personality disorder early on in the engagement process. A personality disorder label has potentially far-reaching consequences and should not be applied in the absence of very thorough and complete information. Therefore, this client's entry would, most properly be entered as follows:

Obsessive Compulsive Personality traits.

Diagnosis deferred (F99)

Rule-out Obsessive-Compulsive Personality Disorder (F60.5)

6. Conduct Disorder, unspecified (F91.9).
NOT INDICATED (-1)

The client's drive to obtain and retain large numbers of items has a flavor of the drive of the impulse control problems (e.g., gambling, stealing, explosive anger, etc.). However, the symptoms that are present are not characteristic of other disruptive, impulse-control or conduct disorders. The client is clearly driven to collect and hoard items, even in the face of great personal cost (e.g., the loss of the use of her home, and other physical space and functional limitations).

RESPONSE DEVELOPMENT:

It would appear that the appropriate provisional diagnosis would be Hoarding Disorder (F42.3) As the client shows obsessive compulsive personality traits, further investigation and multiple visits with the client could help confirm or rule-out obsessive-compulsive personality disorder. The client may also be given the diagnosis "Problems of Adjustment to Life-Cycle Transitions (Z60.0)" due to the multiple aging issues impacting her life. If multiple mental health diagnoses end up existing after subsequent visits, they should be ranked as "primary," "secondary," and "tertiary," according to the severity of their impact on the client, the more fundamental (root of) problem (e.g., depression, secondary to frequently alcohol use), and/or the focus of treatment—as per agency and/or insurance guidelines.

This page is intentionally blank.

Section D: Based on the transitional, provisional diagnosis, identify appropriate treatment methods for this situation.

DIRECTIONS: Select as many as you consider indicated in this Section. After making your selections and scoring your answers, it is beneficial to read the rationales and extended scenarios for all answer choices.

☐ 1. Cognitive Behavioral Therapy.
☐ 2. Group Therapy.
☐ 3. Gestalt Therapy.
☐ 4. Exposure and Response Prevention (ERP) Therapy.
☐ 5. Dream analysis to explore repressed subconscious issues.
☐ 6. Serotonin Reuptake Inhibitor (SRI) medications.
☐ 7. Anxiolytic medications.
☐ 8. Rational-Emotive Therapy.

Section D: Treatment Approach Relevance and Selection.

1. Cognitive Behavioral Therapy.
INDICATED (+1)

A Cognitive Behavioral approach would be among the most effective for this client's situation. The goal of CBT for hoarding disorder is to decrease clutter via enhanced decision-making and organizational skills, and strengthening the client's resistance to urges to collect and save things. While CBT does not "cure" hoarding disorder, it can significantly decrease the problem in many individuals.

2. Group Therapy.
INDICATED (+1)

While those with Obsessive Compulsive Personality Disorder often do not respond well to group therapy and self-help support groups, individuals with compulsive hoarding tendencies do derive meaningful support and progress via these approaches.

3. Gestalt Therapy.
NOT INDICATED (-1)

Gestalt therapy focuses on experiential processes and on content, with an emphasis on thoughts, feelings, and actions in the present moment. It uses a technique called "mindfulness" to link direct experience and indirect or secondary interpretations. There is no indication that Gestalt Therapy has been helpful to clients dealing with compulsive hoarding.

4. Exposure and Response Prevention (ERP) Therapy.
INDICATED (+2)

ERP treatment involves retraining behavior patterns. Those with hoarding disorder are encouraged to resist compulsive hoarding behaviors such as postponing decisions, saving things "just in case," and piling things instead of storing them. They are gradually exposed to behaviors such as throwing things away, storing things, and organizing things effectively. This ultimately changes the way people with hoarding disorder think and behave in relation to their possessions.

5. Dream analysis to explore repressed subconscious issues.
NOT INDICATED (-2)

Dream analysis has not effective relationship to hoarding disorder.

6. Serotonin Reuptake Inhibitor (SRI) medications.
INDICATED (+2)

While controversial, SRI medications are believed to be effective in reducing hoarding disorder behaviors in some individuals – particularly when combined with cognitive-behavioral approaches such as Exposure and Response Prevention (ERP), and support groups, etc.

7. Anxiolytic medications.
NOT INDICATED (-1)

While some measure of anxiety is experienced by compulsive hoarders, especially when confronted with throwing out worn-out and unneeded items, anxiolytic medications have not demonstrated any efficacy in treating this disorder.

8. Rational-Emotive Therapy (RET).
NOT INDICATED (-2)

There is no information indicating that RET would be effective in treating hoarding disorder.

SUMMARY:

The tendency toward hoarding disorders appears to arise from a combination of situational and even genetic factors (it appears to run in families). While treatment is difficult, and progress takes considerable time (and while the tendency is never extinguished entirely), a combination of Cognitive-Behavioral Therapy (such as Exposure and Response Prevention) combined with group therapy strategies, as well as Serotonin Reuptake Inhibitor medications has some supporting evidence.

SCORING: (Max = maximum possible; MPL = minimum passing level)

6A. Max 10; MPL 7
6B. Max 10; MPL 7
6C. Max 3; MPL 2
6D. Max 6; MPL 4

This page is intentionally blank.

Simulation #7

As a psychiatric consultant for a county jail facility, you were called to evaluate an inmate for possible alcoholism and withdrawal symptoms. Tony was a 42-year-old advertising executive who was arrested for driving under the influence (DUI). His Highway Patrol-administered breathalyzer test estimated his blood alcohol level to be 0.09%—just slightly over the 0.08% limit in his state. He did not manage to produce bail, as the accident resulted in injuries and a commensurately high bond. He was contesting the arrest, and was incarcerated for some 36 hours. Jail staff noted that his hands seemed to be tremulous, and he presented as agitated, irritable, and moody. Concerned that his symptoms might escalate, you were called to evaluate his situation.

NOW GO TO SECTION A.

Section A: Initial Information Gathering.

Given the information provided, which of the following would be important in formulating a provisional DSM diagnosis?

DIRECTIONS: Select as many as you consider correct. After making your selections and scoring your answers, it is beneficial to read the rationales and extended scenarios for all answer choices.

- ☐ 1. Medical history.
- ☐ 2. Employment history.
- ☐ 3. Alcohol abuse history.
- ☐ 4. Educational history.
- ☐ 5. Psychiatric history.
- ☐ 6. Substance abuse history.
- ☐ 7. Current prescription medications.
- ☐ 8. Legal history.

NOW GO TO SECTION B.

Section A: Relevance and Initial Information Obtained.

1. Medical history.
INDICATED (+2)

The client indicates that he has been diagnosed with "essential tremor"—a neurological disorder of unknown etiology that produces involuntary shaking, especially of the hands. Thus, he dismissed the reports of jail staff and insisted that they had simply overlooked his condition earlier—adding that it was probably not as noticeable when he was intoxicated.

2. Employment history.
NOT INDICATED (-1)

This information would not contribute to the determination of a presenting diagnosis.

3. Alcohol abuse history.
INDICATED (+2)

The client confirms a history of alcohol use, but insists that he is normally only a moderate drinker—a glass of wine at dinner, and a nightcap just prior to retiring to bed. Therefore, he insists, he could not be experiencing alcohol withdrawal symptoms. When asked about his recent episode of intoxication, he clarifies that he had been at a business dinner, and had simply overlooked drinking a third glass of wine prior to his departure for home.

4. Educational history.
NOT INDICATED (-1)

The client's educational history would not be relevant to a presenting diagnosis.

5. Psychiatric history.
INDICATED (+2)

The client denies any past psychiatric history—specifically, that he has never been seen psychiatrically in the past, that he has no past history of psychiatric medications, no psychiatric hospitalizations, and no other psychiatric symptoms in his past. He admits only to the occasional use of Xanax, as prescribed by a physician to treat mild symptoms of anxiety in business and public speaking situations. Pressed further, he admits to having taken this medication just prior to his business meeting, but adamantly denied regular use.

6. Substance abuse history.
INDICATED (+1)

It would be important to know if the client has any other substance use or abuse issues. However, other than moderate social drinking and the episodic use of anxiolytic medications, it does not appear that the client uses any other substances—and none to excess—including prescription and illicit drugs or substances.

7. Current prescription medications.
INDICATED (+2)

This could be important information when considering a presenting diagnosis. However, the client denies the use of any prescription medications beyond the episodic use of an anxiolytic benzodiazepine, Xanax (Alprazolam), as previously noted. The client insists that he takes the medication only as prescribed by his physician, and that the use of this medication is rare.

8. Legal history.
INDICATED (+1)

This information would be useful in determining a presenting diagnosis. However, law enforcement indicates that the client has no prior DUI arrest history, per their records review.

INITIAL FORMULATION:

The client indicated that the tremulousness of his hands was due to a condition called "essential tremor" and not indicative of early withdrawal symptoms. Although jail staff also described the client as "as agitated, irritable, and moody," these symptoms were not overtly evident during your contact. Indeed, beyond what seemed to be somewhat pressured speech, the client's emotional and physical presentation seemed within reasonable parameters given the situation. His claim of "moderate" drinking seemed in line with the Dietary Guidelines for Americans, as released by the U.S. Department of Health and Human Services and the U.S. Department of Agriculture in 2015. They indicated that "moderate alcohol consumption" would consist of "up to one drink per day for women and up to two drinks per day for men" (with a drink defined as 12 oz. of regular beer, 5 oz. of wine (12% alcohol), or 1.5 oz. of 80-proof distilled spirits)—though many experts insist that any "daily" consumption of alcohol breeches the "moderate use" definition. Benzodiazepine withdrawal can mimic the symptoms of alcohol withdrawal. However, the client denied excessive use of his prescription anxiolytic, Xanax. Knowing the importance of quality collateral contacts, and to further confirm the client's story, you obtain an information release to speak with his prescribing physician, as well as his spouse, Vicky.

This page is intentionally blank.

Section B:

ADDITIONAL INFORMATION: It was now into the weekend, so contact with the client's physician was not immediately possible (though a message was left with his message exchange). However, the client's wife was contacted that same evening. When pressed, she admitted that the client seemed to be "drinking more than usual lately," but she seemed reluctant to discuss this further. She did, however, clarify that "lately" would be the last few months, not just days or weeks. One day later, contact was made with the client's prescribing physician for the Xanax. At the outset the physician denied that the client had a diagnosis of "essential tremor" or "any other neurological disorder" that he was aware of or had observed. Further, he noted having been recently contacted by another physician who was also seeing the client for "issues of anxiety," and who was also prescribing the client Xanax. The physician pointed out that there could be other sources beyond himself and the second doctor. Therefore, he could not be certain how much the client was abusing benzodiazepines.

Based on all available data, identify the most appropriate presenting diagnosis for this client:

DIRECTIONS: Select the most appropriate initial diagnosis, given the available information. Check your answer. If your answer is not the one indicated write down your point value, then choose another answer and check your score again. Your score from this section will be the numbers added together. (For example: If your first choice was not indicated and had a score of -1, and your second answer choice was the one indicated with a score of +3, your score for this section would be a +2.)

- ☐ 1. Alcohol Abuse, uncomplicated (F10.10).
- ☐ 2. Sedative, Hypnotic or Anxiolytic Abuse, uncomplicated (F13.10).
- ☐ 3. Alcohol Use, unspecified with Alcohol-Induced Mood Disorder (F10.94).
- ☐ 4. Sedative, Hypnotic or Anxiolytic Use, unspecified with Sedative, Hypnotic or Anxiolytic-Induced Mood Disorder (F13.94).
- ☐ 5. Alcohol Dependence with Withdrawal, unspecified (F10.239).
- ☐ 6. Sedative, Hypnotic, or Anxiolytic Dependence Withdrawal, unspecified (F13.239).
- ☐ 7. Illness, unspecified (R69).

NOW GO TO SECTION C.

Section B: Relevance of Diagnostic Options Presented.

1. Alcohol Abuse, uncomplicated (F10.10).
NOT INDICATED (-1)

The client has experienced an arrest secondary to his use of alcohol. However, the criteria for alcohol-related use disorder requires recurrent (i.e., multiple episodes of arrests or other maladaptive events secondary to use of the substance). Yet, there is no evidence that he has been failing in his work or relationships, or that he has repeatedly been putting himself or others at risk by driving while intoxicated (indeed, the client specifically denies this), or that there are other persistent problems due to abuse of the substance.

2. Sedative, Hypnotic or Anxiolytic Abuse, uncomplicated (F13.10).
NOT INDICATED (-1)

As noted above, the client has experienced an arrest secondary to his use of alcohol. Although he indicated he frequently uses the benzodiazepine known as Xanax, he denies it was used at the time of his arrest. Even "doctor hopping" for prescriptions is insufficient to prove abuse of this substance. The criteria for substance use disorder cannot be met without recurrent episodes of arrests or other maladaptive events. There is no evidence that he has been failing in his work or relationships, or that he has repeatedly been putting himself or others at risk by driving while under the influence of this pharmaceutical medication (indeed, the client specifically denies recent use), or that there are other persistent problems due to abuse of the substance.

3. Alcohol Use, unspecified with Alcohol-Induced Mood Disorder (F10.94).
NOT INDICATED (-1)

Jail staff had described the client as "as agitated, irritable, and moody." Clearly, the client had also been drinking. However, these symptoms were not overtly evident during your contact, and there was as yet no evidence that alcohol was "etiologically related to the disturbance."

4. Sedative, Hypnotic or Anxiolytic Use, unspecified with Sedative, Hypnotic or Anxiolytic-Induced Mood Disorder (F13.94).
NOT INDICATED (-1)

The client was described by jail staff as "as agitated, irritable, and moody." Further, the client had acknowledged use of prescription anxiolytic mediations. However, he denied use on the day of his arrest. Further, these symptoms were not overtly evident during your contact, and there was as yet no evidence that his Xanax was "etiologically related to the disturbance."

5. Alcohol Dependence with Withdrawal, unspecified (F10.239).
NOT INDICATED (-1)

The client acknowledges the moderate alcohol consumption. However, he specifically denies regular excessive use. Further, other essential features of withdrawal are absent: The client denies heavy or prolonged alcohol consumption, so Criteria A can't be met. At the time of your visit two or more of the suggested signs of withdrawal are not present. And finally, per the client, his use of alcohol is not interfering with social and occupational functioning. Unless the client showed actual physical symptoms of withdrawal you cannot infer his alcohol consumption amount and timeline at this time without further information.

6. Sedative, Hypnotic, or Anxiolytic Dependence Withdrawal, unspecified (F13.239).
NOT INDICATED (-1)

The client acknowledges the use of the prescription anxiolytic Xanax. However, he specifically denies regular use. Further, other essential features of withdrawal are absent: The exact length of time the patient has been using the drug is unknown, so Criteria A can't be met. At the time of your visit two or more of the suggested signs of withdrawal are not present. And finally, per the client, his use of anxiolytics is not interfering with social and occupational functioning.

7. Illness, unspecified (R69).
INDICATED (+3)

This would be the most appropriate initial diagnosis, given all available information and the patient's current presentation. While one might be tempted to assign a diagnosis of Alcohol Dependence with Intoxication, unspecified(F10.229), this would not be appropriate as it applies only when the intoxication is current.

ADDITIONAL INFORMATION: Within the next 12 hours, the client's presentation deteriorated further. His tremulousness increased, he became sweaty and tachycardic (pulse above 100 bpm), and he seemed episodically agitated, confused and anxious. Further, at times he seemed responsive to visual and/or auditory hallucinations, as he appeared to make comments to people or voices not in evidence to those around him. Fearful that his situation was worsening, you were again called. Arriving shortly, you confirmed all of the above information.

This page is intentionally blank.

Section C: Provisional Diagnosis Formulation.

Based upon all available information, what would appear to be the most appropriate primary and secondary provisional diagnoses?

DIRECTIONS: Select the TWO most appropriate options provided in this section. Check your answers. If your answers are not the ones indicated, write down your point value, then choose another answer and check your score again. Your score from this section will be the scores of all of your selections added together.

- □ 1. Alcohol Dependence with Alcohol-Induced Psychotic Disorder with Hallucinations (F10.951).
- □ 2. Alcohol Dependence with Withdrawal Delirium (F10.231).
- □ 3. Alcohol Abuse, uncomplicated (F10.10).
- □ 4. Alcohol Dependence with Withdrawal, unspecified (F10.239).
- □ 5. Sedative, Hypnotic, or Anxiolytic Use, unspecified, uncomplicated (F13.90).
- □ 6. Sedative, Hypnotic or Anxiolytic Dependence with Withdrawal Delirium (F13.231).
- □ 7. Sedative, Hypnotic or Anxiolytic Dependence with Other Sedative, Hypnotic or Anxiolytic-Induced Disorder (F13.288).
- □ 8. Brief Psychotic Disorder (F23).

NOW GO TO SECTION D.

Section C: Potential Relevance and Diagnostic Formulation.

1. Alcohol Dependence with Alcohol-Induced Psychotic Disorder with Hallucinations (F10.951).

NOT INDICATED (-1)

The DSM notes: "This diagnosis should be made...only when the symptoms of delusions or hallucinations dominate the clinical picture and are sufficiently severe to warrant independent clinical attention." The client's psychotic symptoms are common in circumstances of alcohol withdrawal, and do not "warrant independent clinical attention," as they do not put the client's life and well-being at undue risk, and will concurrently resolve when appropriate treatment is provided.

2. Alcohol Dependence with Withdrawal Delirium (F10.231).

NOT INDICATED (-1)

The DSM notes: "This diagnosis should be made...only when the cognitive symptoms are in excess of those usually associated with the withdrawal syndrome and when the symptoms are sufficiently severe to warrant independent clinical attention." The client's symptoms of delirium are common in circumstances of alcohol withdrawal, and do not "warrant independent clinical attention" as they do not put the client's life and well-being at undue risk, and will concurrently resolve when appropriate treatment is provided.

3. Alcohol Abuse, uncomplicated (F10.10).

INDICATED – SECONDARY DIAGNOSIS (+3)

The client does meet criteria for "Alcohol Use Disorder," as he is 1) showing signs of withdrawal, 2) his drinking has been increasing (per wife), 3) important social/occupational/recreational activities have been impacted, and 4) alcohol continues to be used in spite of negative consequences. Only three are required for this diagnosis. However, the clinical focus at this time would be on the client's withdrawal symptoms – particularly given the dangers involved if the withdrawal symptoms worsen (e.g., they could become life-threatening). Therefore, this would not be the "primary" diagnosis, but rather the secondary diagnosis.

4. Alcohol Withdrawal (F10.239).

INDICATED – PRIMARY DIAGNOSIS (+3)

The client's withdrawal symptoms now suggest that Criterion A has been met (heavy and prolonged drinking). Further, five of the eight items under Criteria B have also been met – 1) autonomic hyperactivity; 2) increased hand tremor; 3) "transient visual, tactile, or auditory hallucinations or illusions"; 4) psychomotor agitation; and 5) anxiety. Only two are required to meet the diagnostic threshold. Finally, the symptoms found in Criterion B have resulted in "clinically significant distress or impairment in social, occupational, or other important areas of functioning," and "the symptoms are not due to a general medical condition and are not better accounted for by another mental disorder."

5. Sedative, Hypnotic, or Anxiolytic Use, unspecified, uncomplicated (F13.90).

NOT INDICATED (-1)

There is insufficient evidence to warrant the application of this diagnosis. The client's anxiolytic use does appear to be problematic. It is even possible, given that benzodiazepines are a first-line treatment for alcohol withdrawal symptoms, that the client is self-medicating using anxiety as an excuse. However, in the absence of more definitive information, this diagnosis cannot be reliably applied.

6. Sedative, Hypnotic or Anxiolytic Dependence with Withdrawal Delirium (F13.231).
NOT INDICATED (-1)

As with Anxiolytic Use Disorder, there is insufficient evidence to warrant the application of this diagnosis.

7. Sedative, Hypnotic or Anxiolytic Dependence with Other Sedative, Hypnotic or Anxiolytic-Induced Disorder (F13.288).
NOT INDICATED (-1)

Not only is there insufficient evidence of the duration and intensity of the client's anxiolytic use, it is not advisable to apply an unspecified diagnostic label when a more definitive option exists.

8. Brief Psychotic Disorder (F23).
NOT INDICATED (-1)

This diagnosis is only used when the psychotic symptoms in evidence are "not due to the direct physiological effects of a substance (e.g., a drug of abuse, a medication) or a general medical condition." In this case, "a substance" (alcohol) better explains the client's apparent hallucinations.

This page is intentionally blank.

Section D: Decision Making

DIRECTIONS: Select as many appropriate early interventions as you consider indicated at this point. After making your selections and scoring your answers, it is beneficial to read the rationales and extended scenarios for all answer choices.

- ☐ 1. Providing the client with a minimum amount of alcohol to help control his escalating withdrawal symptoms.
- ☐ 2. Psychiatric hospitalization.
- ☐ 3. Immediate medical hospitalization.
- ☐ 4. Immediate physician referral to obtain treatment for the client's escalating withdrawal symptoms.
- ☐ 5. Biofeedback, involving either audio or visual feedback, to control the client's agitation and other withdrawal symptoms.
- ☐ 6. Confront the client candidly and directly regarding his prior denials of "heavy" alcohol and anxiolytic use and abuse.
- ☐ 7. Secure drug and alcohol toxicology testing.
- ☐ 8. Encourage the client to fully disclose the extent of his alcohol and prescription drug use to ensure full and timely treatment.

NOW GO TO SECTION E.

Section D: Options Relevance and Findings.

1. Providing the client with a minimum amount of alcohol to help control his escalating withdrawal symptoms.
NOT INDICATED (-2)

This intervention would be highly counter-productive. It could potentially reinforce continued alcohol use, it merely delays the withdrawal recovery process, and it cannot be reliably administered ("dosage" questions cannot be readily or properly addressed).

2. Psychiatric hospitalization.
NOT INDICATED (-1)

The client's immediate problem – alcohol withdrawal – requires an immediate medical intervention, rather than a primarily psychiatric approach. Therefore, psychiatric hospitalization would not be indicated.

3. Immediate medical hospitalization.
NOT INDICATED (-1)

Alcohol withdrawal can normally be successfully treated on an outpatient basis. Thus, inpatient medical hospitalization would not be indicated.

4. Immediate physician referral to obtain treatment for the client's escalating withdrawal symptoms.
INDICATED (+3)

It is essential that the client be referred to a physician for treatment of his escalating alcohol withdrawal symptoms. While the extent of his alcohol abuse remains unknown (the wife indicates only his increased consumption of alcohol over the past few months), it is essential that the withdrawal symptoms not be permitted to progress into what might become a life-threatening situation (e.g., potential grand mal seizures, etc.).

5. Biofeedback, involving either audio or visual feedback, to control the client's agitation and other withdrawal symptoms.
NOT INDICATED (-1)

Biofeedback in any form would not be indicated for the primary management of withdrawal symptoms associated with substance abuse.

6. Confront the client candidly and directly regarding his prior denials of "heavy" alcohol and anxiolytic use and abuse.
NOT INDICATED (-1)

Collateral information from the client's spouse and prescribing physician has revealed that the client has not been forthright about the extent of his alcohol and benzodiazepine abuse. At some point, these issues will need to be addressed. This, however, must first await treatment of the client's withdrawal symptoms. Confrontation prematurely, particularly when the client is cognitively and physiologically compromised, would not be productive.

7. Secure drug and alcohol toxicology testing.
NOT INDICATED (-1)

The client received a blood alcohol test shortly after his arrest, at his insistence that he was not over the legal limit. However, the results of this test are still pending. Further testing for the blood level of alcohol would be fruitless, as it is metabolized out of the body within 3-10 hours. Although heavy use of benzodiazepines can be detected via toxicology screening for a period of up to six weeks, it is not an illicit drug and successful treatment requires client candor and cooperation. Further, withdrawal from benzodiazepines is not life-threatening, and therefore, blood testing is not requisite medically. Therefore, securing testing for this pharmaceutical medication would not be indicated.

8. Encourage the client to fully disclose the extent of his alcohol and prescription drug use to ensure full and timely treatment.
INDICATED (+1)

Clients should always be thoughtfully and supportively encouraged to disclose the full extent of their alcohol and substance use in order to meaningfully further the treatment process.

This page is intentionally blank.

Section E: Based on the secondary diagnosis above, identify appropriate short-term treatment goals for this client.

DIRECTIONS: Select appropriate short-term treatment goals from among the following. After making your selections and scoring your answers, it is beneficial to read the rationales and extended scenarios for all answer choices.

- ☐ 1. Ongoing participation in an Alcoholics Anonymous or similar program.
- ☐ 2. Participation in Narc-Anon for additional support.
- ☐ 3. Family participation in Al-Anon.
- ☐ 4. Identification of "triggers" that lead to drinking.
- ☐ 5. Involvement in calming imagery and relaxation exercises.
- ☐ 6. Enrollment in an educational program for career advancement.

Section E: Treatment Goal Relevance and Rationale.

1. Ongoing participation in an Alcoholics Anonymous or similar program.
INDICATED (+2)

12-step programs such as Alcoholics Anonymous have a remarkable track record for motivating individuals to become and stay sober. Participation in AA or a similar 12-step program would be an excellent short-term and long-term goal for this client.

2. Participation in Narc-Anon for additional support.
NOT INDICATED (-1)

Narc-Anon is a recovery program for narcotics addicts, and does not offer services specific to alcohol recovery. Given that the client has no narcotics addition issues, participation in Narc-Anon would not be an appropriate short-term (or long-term) treatment goal.

3. Family participation in Al-Anon.
INDICATED (+2)

The client is married and has three children. Al-Anon is specifically designed to help family members cope with, support, and facilitate recovery for individuals with a drinking problem. Referring the family to Al-Anon would be an important short-term goal for this client and his family.

4. Identification of "triggers" that lead to drinking.
INDICATED (+1)

Addictive behaviors are accompanied by "triggers" that motivate individuals to engage in their addiction. Identifying key triggers that motivate this client to drink, as well as identifying alternatives and better coping skills, would be very positive short-term treatment goals.

5. Involvement in calming imagery and relaxation exercises.
INDICATED (+1)

The client has indicated that he struggles with feelings of anxiety, and that these feelings lead to substance use (both drinking and anxiolytic use). Engaging the client in developing calming imagery and relaxation exercises would therefore be a positive short-term goal.

6. Enrollment in an educational program for career advancement.
NOT INDICATED (-1)

There is no information suggesting that the client needs to train for a new career. Therefore, this would not be a meaningful short-term goal for this client.

SCORING: (Max = maximum possible; MPL = minimum passing level)

7A. Max 10; MPL 8
7B. Max 3; MPL 2
7C. Max 6; MPL 5
7D. Max 4; MPL 3
7E. Max 6; MPL 4

Simulation #8

You are an Employee Assistance Program (EAP) counselor at a large health care facility. A 32-year-old male nurse, Richard, is referred to you by his supervisor. The referral indicates that he is an ICU nurse, and that he has been "highly volatile" with angry outbursts in the ICU, at times with patients and family members, but primarily with co-workers. You are requested to evaluate his situation, assist him with anger management, and report on his fitness for continued assignment in that high-stress setting.

NOW GO TO SECTION A.

Section A: Initial Information Gathering.

Select the questions that would be useful in learning more about this client's insight into his anger management issues.

DIRECTIONS: Select as many as you consider indicated in this section. After making your selections and scoring your answers, it is beneficial to read the rationales and extended scenarios for all answer choices.

- ☐ 1. His understanding of the purpose of the referral.
- ☐ 2. What he hopes to accomplish through counseling.
- ☐ 3. His continuing education plans.
- ☐ 4. His belief about what caused his emotional outbursts.
- ☐ 5. The extent and quality of his relational support system.
- ☐ 6. How long he has been assigned to the ICU setting.
- ☐ 7. If he has a current or past history of substance abuse.
- ☐ 8. The stability of his financial circumstances.

NOW GO TO SECTION B.

Section A: Element Relevance and Initial Information Obtained.

1. His understanding of the purpose of the referral.
INDICATED (+2)

The client's perception of the purpose for the referral is important. When questioned, the client properly expresses an understanding that he is there to address issues of angry outbursts in the workplace.

2. What he hopes to accomplish through counseling.
INDICATED (+2)

This is a meaningful, open-ended question. The client states that he would like to gain control over his anger in order to become a better, calmer, and more dependable employee.

3. His continuing education plans.
NOT INDICATED (-1)

The client's continuing education plans are not relevant to revealing his "insight into his anger management issues."

4. His belief about what caused his emotional outbursts.
INDICATED (+1)

This question could reveal a great deal about the client's insight into his anger management issues.

5. The extent and quality of his relational support system.
INDICATED (+1)

The extent and kinds of relational supports that the client has maintained can aid in determining his capacity to relate well with others, which can then be used to better appreciate his insight and understanding into his anger issues. Although the client moved to the area about three years previously, he has yet to establish meaningful relationships with more than a very few others – and these are more casual in nature (i.e., neighbors, coworkers, friends of his spouse, etc., that he does not describe as "close" in any way to him). He explained that he escaped a drug abuse history during the last 4-6 years prior to relocating. Entering a rehabilitation program, he cut social ties with his past, as directed, in order to remain "clean and sober." He is married to his third wife – the other two left him during his drug use years. He speaks highly of his current spouse of 5 years. She is a Filipino woman (from the Philippines), new to the United States, who also cares for her aged parents in their home.

6. How long he has been assigned to the ICU setting.
NOT INDICATED (-1)

While it may be incidentally useful to know the length of time the client has been in his current work setting, it will not be immediately useful in determining his insight into his angry outburst problems.

7. If he has a current or past history of substance abuse.
INDICATED (+2)

Poor emotional control is often both a precursor to and a persistent problem with substance abusers (whether using alcohol or drugs), as it is a way for them to alleviate their distress, retreat from reality, and, sometimes, to act out emotionally with less accountability (e.g., "I was drunk when I did that; I didn't mean anything by it"). The client states that he has been drug and alcohol free for about seven years. Prior to that time he drank heavily and episodically ingested both cocaine (free-based) and methamphetamines (smoked).

8. The stability of his financial circumstances.
NOT INDICATED (-1)

The client's current financial circumstances may be of some incidental value, but this information will not shed light on his anger management issues.

ADDITIONAL INFORMATION: In conversation with the referring supervisor, you learn the following: 1) the client has been disciplined ("written up") for being overly rough in moving and treating his patients, for angrily shouting at others in sudden outbursts, and for intimidating others by means of aggressive posture, threatening gestures, loud verbal remonstrations, episodic use of foul language, and stalking out during essential work discussions; 2) the client has been resistive to counsel and direction—especially when offered by women administrators; 3) the client has been perceived by others as reluctant to share in patient care (e.g., moving patients when a two-person lift is required, cross-covering during lunch breaks, etc.); and 4) the client is perceived as very "short-fused" and very blaming of others if things don't go as he had expected. He is also a "large, muscular, stocky man who easily appears intimidating to others."

This page is intentionally blank.

Section B: Based upon all available information, identify additional issues needing to be addressed.

DIRECTIONS: Select as many as seem correct and necessary. After making your selections and scoring your answers, it is beneficial to read the rationales and extended scenarios for all answer choices.

- ☐ 1. Explore the client current marital issues.
- ☐ 2. Evaluate professional training needs.
- ☐ 3. Inquire about his efforts to remain clean and sober (e.g., AA attendance, counseling, work with an addiction counselor and/or AA "sponsor").
- ☐ 4. Delve into his feelings about working in a stressful of an ICU setting.
- ☐ 5. Address his feelings about working in a women-dominated profession.
- ☐ 6. Discuss his communication style.
- ☐ 7. Review his style of dealing with confrontation and disagreements.
- ☐ 8. Examine his feelings about accepting supervision and direction.

NOW GO TO SECTION C.

Section B: Relevance of Potential Information Needing Address.

1. Explore the client current marital issues.
NOT INDICATED (-1)

There is no indication that the client has active marital issues. He speaks "highly" of his spouse, and has not indicated that there are problems at home. It is worthy of note, however, that he has married a first-generation (foreign-born) Asian woman some eight years his junior (at age 24 she is the youngest in a large family, and is caring for her aged parents), and from a culture that permits higher levels of male dominance than does the client's native culture.

2. Evaluate professional training needs.
NOT INDICATED (-2)

There is no indication that the client has professional training issues (i.e., in terms of his medical nursing practice), and therefore, it should not be presumed.

3. Inquire about his efforts to remain clean and sober (e.g., AA attendance, counseling, work with an addiction counselor and/or AA "sponsor").
INDICATED (+2)

Given the client's statement that he has a history of drug and alcohol abuse, it is important to inquire about his efforts at remaining clean and sober. The client states that he has become irregular in his AA attendance, but that he does go "when the need arises," and that he has an established a relationship with a sponsor since he moved into the area.

4. Delve into his feelings about working in a stressful of an ICU setting.
INDICATED (+2)

Work in an ICU setting is particularly demanding and stressful. In exploring the client's feelings about working in a less arduous setting, the client responded, "I'm either an ICU nurse or an ER nurse, or nothing at all. I will never work in a regular 'floor care' setting or in a clinic office. That's not me. I work ICU or ER only, and that's all I'll accept."

5. Address his feelings about working in a women-dominated profession.
INDICATED (+1)

It is clear that he has difficulty working with women. However, he does not acknowledge this, saying that he has no problem working with women in any capacity.

6. Discuss his communication style.
INDICATED (+1)

The client is reportedly clipped and intolerant in dealing with others, and walks out on staff, patients, and their families if he does not agree with them. When this is addressed, the client refuses responsibility for any such past incidents, indicating only that he has no obligation to tolerate "lectures" from anyone.

7. Review his style of dealing with confrontation and disagreements.
INDICATED (+1)

The client is unwilling to work out disagreements. However, when this was gently suggested, the client indicated that "quibbling" was a "waste of time" and that he wasn't obliged to participate—even with a "charge nurse" during a work shift.

8. Examine his feelings about accepting supervision and direction.
INDICATED (+2)

The client not only refuses to relinquish control to his coworkers, but to supervisory staff as well. In addressing this, the client indicated that he was only obliged to "kowtow" to administrative staff, to whom shift supervisors and charge nurse staff also report. He emphasized that lower level leaders were just "glorified line staff," and that he had no obligation to take direction from them.

ADDITIONAL INFORMATION: In reviewing his past drug and alcohol use, at least seven years in the past, the client noted that he "ran with a rough crowd." Frequenting bars and other high-conflict settings, he also frequently engaged in fighting. On one occasion, he was in a "knife fight" with a man that he believed died from the event. "I stuck my knife in his neck, and when I pulled back, his blood spurted all over. I can't imagine that he could have possibly survived." He then asked you to keep this revelation confidential. When asked if his involvement in the incident ever became known, he said, "We all took off long before the police arrived, and no one ever talked to me about it again."

This page is intentionally blank.

Section C: Ethical Decision Making.

Given the client's stated involvement in the deliberate violent death of another human being, choose the best response from the options that follow.

DIRECTIONS: Select the best response available in this section. Check your answer. If your answer is not the one indicated write down your point value, then choose another answer and check your score again. Your score from this section will be the numbers added together. (For example: If your first choice was not indicated and had a score of -1, and your second answer choice was the one indicated with a score of +3, your score for this section would be a +2.)

- ☐ 1. Contact local law enforcement and report the client's revelation.
- ☐ 2. Contact a lawyer and discuss your legal and ethical obligations in this situation.
- ☐ 3. Review what you have learned with another consulting mental health professional to obtain proper guidance.
- ☐ 4. Call the local Adult Protective Services agency, in keeping with "Tarasoff" directives, so that they can lodge criminal charges against the client.
- ☐ 5. Place the client on an involuntary hold, due to his self-proclaimed danger to others.
- ☐ 6. Address the disclosure only in terms of exploring his aggressive tendencies, and not in terms of any legal or ethical response to the past event.
- ☐ 7. Contact the referring administrator, and report his dangerous behavior.
- ☐ 8. Report your concerns to the hospital's Ethics Committee, which will then take whatever action is necessary.

NOW GO TO SECTION D.

Section C: Relevance of the option chosen.

1. Contact local law enforcement and report the client's revelation.
NOT INDICATED (-1)

Counselors are directed to contact law enforcement only for disclosures that involve: 1) threats of violence to others (directly or indirectly); 2) situations of child abuse, no matter how distant, if the victim is still a minor; 3) situations of elder abuse (in some states); and/or 4) situations of dependent adult abuse (in some states). All other crimes do not involve mandatory reporting. Consult your local laws regarding situations 3 and 4, above.

2. Contact a lawyer and discuss your legal and ethical obligations in this situation.
NOT INDICATED (-1)

Given that distant crimes, involving circumstances as enumerated above, are not subject to mandatory reporting, no legal consultation is required. In circumstances where a moral obligation to report may exist, careful legal consultation is required to avoid potential legal liability via breach of confidentiality.

3. Review what you have learned with another consulting mental health professional to obtain proper guidance.
NOT INDICATED (-1)

As noted previously, a crime this remote to the point of disclosure is not subject to mandatory reporting. Disclosures that may confer a moral obligation to report should receive careful consultation before any disclosure to avoid potential legal liability via breach of confidentiality. Obviously, it is incumbent upon the counselor to do all that he/she can to motivate a client toward change and/or self-disclosure, if it is essential, and in the client's and others' best interests.

4. Call the local Adult Protective Services agency, in keeping with "Tarasoff" directives, so that they can lodge criminal charges against the client.
NOT INDICATED (-1)

Adult Protective Services agencies exist to protect elderly and dependent adults in circumstances of recent, ongoing, and/or planned abuse. This situation does not involve any current event, nor does it involve and elderly or dependent adult. Tarasoff statutes dictate that a known potential victim be notified of likely danger or threats of harm, either directly, or indirectly (through another) if no direct mode of contact is possible. This situation does not constitute a current or planned threat of harm to another, and therefore, does not fall under Tarasoff regulations.

5. Place the client on an involuntary hold, due to his self-proclaimed danger to others.
NOT INDICATED (-2)

A client must pose a known and immediate threat to himself or others to be placed on an involuntary hold. In this situation, there is not such immediate threat.

6. Address the disclosure only in terms of exploring his aggressive tendencies, and not in terms of any legal or ethical response to the past event.
INDICATED (+3)

The disclosure was serious, and it should be meaningfully addressed. However, in this therapeutic situation, it reflects primarily upon the client's past history of aggression as it relates to continued aggressive tendencies. Thus, this should be fully explored from this perspective.

7. Contact the referring administrator and report his dangerous behavior.
NOT INDICATED (-1)

The client's disclosure does not constitute currently dangerous behavior. Any such disclosure of this issue would constitute a serious and unethical breach of confidentiality. Indeed, the client has specifically indicated the need for this to remain confidential. Therefore, disclosure by the therapist to the administrator, or anyone else, without the client's explicit permission, would not be permitted.

8. Report your concerns to the hospital's Ethics Committee, who will then take whatever action is necessary.
NOT INDICATED (-2)

Hospital or medical ethics committees exist to assist patients, family, and staff with medical treatment dilemmas. They are not designed to cope with criminal allegations, etc. Further, confidentiality standards prevent disclosing information of this nature without a client's specific written permission, which he has not provided. Therefore, no such disclosure is warranted, appropriate, or possible.

This page is intentionally blank.

Section D: Provisional Diagnosis Formulation.

Based upon the available information, what would appear to be the most appropriate provisional diagnosis for this client?

DIRECTIONS: Select the TWO most appropriate options provided in this Section. Check your answers. If your answers are not the ones indicated, write down your point value, then choose another answer and check your score again. Your score from this section will be the scores of all of your selections added together.

- □ 1. Conduct Disorder, Adolescent onset type (F91.2).
- □ 2. Adjustment Disorder, With Mixed Disturbance of Emotions and Conduct (F43.25).
- □ 3. Intermittent Explosive Disorder (F63.81).
- □ 4. Post-Traumatic Stress Disorder (F43.10).
- □ 5. Dissocial (Antisocial) Personality Disorder (F60.2).
- □ 6. Oppositional Defiant Disorder (F91.3).
- □ 7. Conduct Disorder, unspecified (F91.9).
- □ 8. Other Conduct Disorders (F91.8)
- □ 9. Adult Antisocial Behavior (Z72.811).
- □ 10. Unspecified Problems Related to Employment (Z56.9)
- □ 11. Social Exclusion or Rejection (Z60.4).

Section D: Relevance and Diagnostic Formulation.

1. Conduct Disorder, Adolescent onset type (F91.2).
NOT INDICATED (-2)

This diagnosis is most often given to adolescents and children. The client does not seem to be currently engaging in violating the rights of others as a whole.

2. Adjustment Disorder, With Mixed Disturbance of Emotions and Conduct (F43.25).
NOT INDICATED (-1).

This diagnosis requires the presence of "identifiable stressor(s)" and the decompensation must have occurred "within 3 months of the onset of the stressor(s)." Given the absence of any specific precipitating stressor(s) – not "triggers" (e.g., contention, etc.), but disturbing stressor(s) – this would not be an appropriate diagnosis.

3. Intermittent Explosive Disorder (F63.81).
NOT INDICATED (-1)

This diagnosis requires "several discrete episodes of failure to resist aggressive impulses that result in serious assaultive acts or destruction of property." Given that no assaults or property destruction has occurred, this would not be an appropriate diagnosis.

4. Post-Traumatic Stress Disorder (F43.10).
NOT INDICATED (-1)

This disorder is predicated upon the witnessing of an event or events that produced emotional trauma. A clear external precipitating event, as well as classic symptoms such as flashbacks, intrusive recollections, nightmares, etc., are not evident in this case scenario.

5. Dissocial (Antisocial) Personality Disorder (F60.2).
NOT INDICATED (-2)

This disorder requires "a pervasive pattern of disregard for and violation of the rights of others occurring since age 15 years," as well as "evidence of Conduct Disorder with onset before age 15 years." However, no evidence of such history is present in this case scenario. Therefore, this would not be an appropriate diagnosis, given the information available. Further, personality disorders could not be ethically given until considerable more contacts have ensued, and considerable more information has been gathered.

6. Oppositional Defiant Disorder (F91.3).
INDICATED (+2)

This is a disorder is often associated with childhood and adolescence, but in this case the client meets criteria for this disorder despite being an adult. The client exhibits 6 of the possible criteria from Criteria A, and readily meets Criteria B and C. To determine if this is a mild, moderate, or severe disorder, it would need to be determined if work is the only area currently affected or if these behaviors are in all settings.

7. Conduct Disorder, unspecified (F91.9).
NOT INDICATED (-1)

This diagnosis is distinguished by a client engaging in "behaviors that may be harmful to themselves or others." Simple arguing, confrontation, and rude behaviors do not rise to this threshold. Examples of the more serious behavioral diagnoses characteristic of this category include kleptomania and pyromania.

8. Other Conduct Disorders. (F91.8).
NOT INDICATED (-1)

The diagnosis of Other Conduct Disorders is typically used for problems that fall short of Disssocial (Antisocial) Personality Disorder. It is frequently applied to children and adolescents, as an onset by age 10 is part of the typical diagnostic criteria. However, there is room for an "Unspecified Onset", and the diagnosis is specifically permitted to be made in those over the age of 18. However, to meet criteria A of the disorder the client must have 3 of the possible 15 criteria present, and this client only has two: bullying and possibly being cruel to others.

9. Adult Antisocial Behavior (Z72.811).
NOT INDICATED (-1)

This code is typically used for less severe diagnostic issues. Further, "antisocial behavior" that qualifies under this diagnostic category must not be better explained by another mental disorder, and does not necessarily follow any precipitating event. Common examples include: stealing, dealing illegal substances, con-artistry, etc., as opposed to violent acts without remorse, etc. While the client's past behavior suggests that this diagnosis may have applied at some prior time, his current issues do not meet threshold criteria.

10. Unspecified Problems Related to Employment (Z56.9).
INDICATED (+2)

This code accommodates any occupational problem. Therefore, it would be appropriate for this client's situation.

11. Social Exclusion or Rejection (Z60.4).
NOT INDICATED (-1)

This code would often be used when there is bullying or teasing toward the client. In this situation, the client is the one who is being sad to be intimidating.

SCORING: (Max = maximum possible; MPL = minimum passing level)

8A. Max 8; MPL 6
8B. Max 9; MPL 7
8C. Max 3; MPL 2
8D. Max 4; MPL 3

This page is intentionally blank.

Simulation #9

You are a Children's Protective Services agency counselor taking a weekend call. You were contacted by the ex-wife of a 42-year-old man named Jerry (the identified client). Divorced five years, Jerry had dropped off the children at her home on a Friday night, after a week-long vacation on a summer houseboat at a local lake. The wife was to keep the children over the weekend. Jerry was to return the next Monday and pick up the four children—ranging in age from 5 to 15—for the second half of his two-week summer vacation with them. He dropped by the next evening to wash some laundry (at her suggestion, as he was out of state from his home). At that time, she noted Jerry was behaving rather bizarrely. He rushed into the house, hurriedly shut the door behind himself, and then began drawing the curtains in the front room. He claimed he was being followed by some sort of clandestine law enforcement group intent on arresting him. When she tried to look outside, he pulled her back saying "it might not be safe." Staying only a few minutes, he hurried out the back door, got into his car, and sped away. Looking outside, she could see nothing. Her questions of you: What is happening, and is he safe to take the minor children for another week?

NOW GO TO SECTION A.

Section A: Initial Information Gathering.

Select the areas that need to be further explored to better understand the client's status, and his capacity to safely take the minor children for a week.

DIRECTIONS: Select as many as you consider indicated in this section. After making your selections and scoring your answers, it is beneficial to read the rationales and extended scenarios for all answer choices.

- ☐ 1. The onset and duration of the cognitive/behavioral changes seen.
- ☐ 2. The client's past psychiatric history.
- ☐ 3. Date of the patient's last medical exam.
- ☐ 4. The patient's level of education.
- ☐ 5. The client's substance abuse history.
- ☐ 6. The client's employment history.
- ☐ 7. Family mental health history.
- ☐ 8. The client's legal history.

NOW GO TO SECTION B.

Section A: Relevance and Initial Information Explored.

1. The onset and duration of the cognitive/behavioral changes seen.
INDICATED (+2)

When questioned further, the wife added further details. Apparently, when Jerry left her home he went to see a mutual friend. There his paranoia continued, and he demanded a change of clothes "for a disguise." That night, he stayed with mutual friends. The husband in that home, a paramedic, indicated he seemed so "disconnected from reality" that they feared for the safety of their own children, and had them spend the night locked in their bedroom. The next day, they drove Jerry everywhere he wanted to go, concerned that he wouldn't be safe driving alone. As they drove, Jerry would point to parking lots full of empty cars at shopping centers and claim that they were all filled with "undercover agents" just waiting to waylay him. When told the cars were empty, he insisted that the "agents" had simply ducked down as they drew near. However, when Jerry returned to the ex-wife's home on Sunday evening, he seemed entirely normal. Therefore, the duration was approximately 48 hours. He first insisted that he had "just been tired," later that he had experienced "a relapse of PTSD," and later still, that he'd experienced a brief reaction to some "Boron" given him during a medical imaging study for cancer (which he suggested he might now have). Given that he now seemed quite normal, the ex-wife was unsure what to think of him taking the children. When she asked the children if their father seemed "okay" during their vacation, they agreed he was fine, with two exceptions: 1) "He spent almost all the time on the phone with his girlfriend"; and 2) the 15-year-old son recalled his father having hurried them home, saying he was a bit worried "because he'd been visiting some 'dangerous people' just before he came to pick us up." Jerry was very angry at her questioning his capacity to take the children and threatened legal action if she kept them from him. It was at this juncture she called Children's Protective Services.

2. The client's past psychiatric history.
INDICATED (+2)

The client received a diagnosis of PTSD shortly after being discharged from active combat duty in the service. Otherwise, the client has no formal psychiatric history. The wife has long felt he might have some measure of hypochondria, as he seemed to have perpetual doctor visits and was always complaining of health problems of one form or another—heart problems, dramatic injuries (e.g., a "broken back" after surfing, etc.), now cancer, etc. She has also been aware that he has a very manipulative nature, and often seeks to project blame on others for anything that goes wrong. Even so, none of this has been professionally diagnosed.

3. Date of the patient's last medical exam.
NOT INDICATED (-1)

Given the fact that the client is relatively young, purportedly healthy, and has no recent history of hospitalizations, etc., this would not normally be considered relevant to the current situation. Even so, the client claimed to have seen a physician at the Veteran's Administration hospital the day he dropped off the children. While the results of various tests were still pending, he had been released without any restrictions, per his statement to the ex-wife.

4. The patient's level of education.
NOT INDICATED (-1)

Not immediately relevant. Even so, the client has a two-year college degree.

5. The client's substance abuse history.
INDICATED (+2)

During the course of their marriage, the ex-wife noted some unexplained expenditures. When she asked Jerry about them, he claimed they were bank withdrawals "to buy drugs." Consequently, she suspects that he does have a drug abuse history. Further, she is also aware that he seems to routinely be on pain medications for one form of injury or another, and he has been seeing a great many different doctors (i.e., "he always has appointments with doctors, but I don't know what they are for as he won't discuss it most of the time"). As a result, she has some concern that he may have a polypharmacy prescription drug abuse problem. Finally, the client has lost approximately 50 lbs in the last six months, for which he offers no explanation. Concerns about the use of an appetite-suppressant drug such as methamphetamine are thus somewhat pronounced.

6. The client's employment history.
NOT INDICATED (-1)

The client's employment history is unlikely to shed much light on his current presentation. The client has been employed by the military for years—originally as a full-time career member of the army, and later in the Army Reserves. He saw active combat duty in Iraq and Afghanistan, where he served as a sniper, and in Army Intelligence as an interrogator. He also received considerable nursing training at one point, and worked episodically as a medic. Since mustering out, the client has worked in the fire-fighting field, and as a paramedic.

7. Family mental health history.
NOT INDICATED (-2)

The family mental health history would not likely have particular bearing on the immediate presenting problem. It would, however, be useful at a later juncture in the evaluation and treatment process. Of note, the client's family has a history of unstable relationships (serial marriages among all siblings, and their father), medical drug-seeking behavior, as well as serial "medical retirements" following various employment experiences. However, there is no formally documented mental health history in the family.

8. The client's legal history.
INDICATED (+1)

The wife is not aware of any specific legal history. However, following the client's divorce, he repeatedly engaged in financial fraud (credit card fraud, mortgage refinance fraud, forgery of her signature, etc.). Once she discovered his actions, she required that her name be taken off the credit cards, the home equity line of credit, etc., but did not press charges.

This page is intentionally blank.

Section B: Based on the early intake data, identify important interventions needed at this time.

DIRECTIONS: Select as many as you consider indicated in this section. After making your selections and scoring your answers, it is beneficial to read the rationales and extended scenarios for all answer choices.

- ☐ 1. Contact with the client (Jerry) to obtain his side of the story.
- ☐ 2. Contact collateral sources (friends that have voiced concerns).
- ☐ 3. Require the client (Jerry) to submit to drug testing.
- ☐ 4. Formally evaluate the client for symptoms of psychosis.
- ☐ 5. Call law enforcement to investigate the client.
- ☐ 6. Set a court date for a legal determination.
- ☐ 7. Remove the children from the home pending further evaluation.
- ☐ 8. Seek a supervisory consult to obtain more specific direction.

NOW GO TO SECTION C.

Section B: Relevance of Potential Information Needing Address.

1. Contact with the client (Jerry) to obtain his side of the story.
INDICATED (+2)

The client refused to meet, and also refused all discussion, stating only, "You'll need to contact my attorney if you want to talk about this any further," yet also refusing to provide an attorney contact number.

2. Contact collateral sources (friends that have voiced concerns).
INDICATED (+2)

The friend from whom he'd requested clothing for purposes of a "disguise" openly acknowledged what had happened. However, there was nothing more that she could add, as he had come and gone so very quickly after she refused to lend him any clothing. The friends with whom he had spent the night initially acknowledged having "some serious concerns," but then refused to offer any details. They then added, "We're friends with both of them, and we don't want to be put in the middle of this."

3. Require the client (Jerry) to submit to drug testing.
NOT INDICATED (-2)

This would require a court order, and time does not permit this.

4. Formally evaluate the client for symptoms of psychosis.
INDICATED (+1)

A face-to-face evaluation would be ideal. However, the client has already refused to meet.

5. Call law enforcement to investigate the client.
NOT INDICATED (-1)

The client's conduct does not constitute criminal behavior; thus, such a request would be refused.

6. Set a court date for a legal determination.
NOT INDICATED (-1)

There is no time to set a court date prior to the father exercising his court-ordered right to have vacation time with his children.

7. Remove the children from the home pending further evaluation.
NOT INDICATED (-2)

There are no allegations that the ex-wife's care of her children is substandard or compromised in any way. Therefore, removing the children from the home would not be indicated.

8. Seek a supervisory consult to obtain more specific direction.
INDICATED (+3)

In this volatile situation, supervisory consultation would be indicated. State laws and obligations vary greatly. It may be determined that the father cannot take the children until he has spoken with

Children's Protective Services staff. This may be arranged at the ex-wife's home for matters of convenience, and to better observe all involved parties—including the father's presentation, the ex-wife's consistency and stability, the condition of the home, etc.

RESPONSE DEVELOPMENT:

The safety of the children is paramount. Allegations of serious concern have been made. A follow-up evaluation may be required.

This page is intentionally blank.

Section C: Additional Information Gathering.

A second call to the client (Jerry) results in his unexpected agreement to meet on the morning of the day he is to pick up the children. Given what has occurred to this juncture, which of the following should be addressed/evaluated at this meeting?

DIRECTIONS: Select as many as you consider indicated in this section. After making your selections and scoring your answers, it is beneficial to read the rationales and extended scenarios for all answer choices.

- ☐ 1. Administration of the Folstein Mini-Mental Status Evaluation.
- ☐ 2. Direct questions about substance abuse.
- ☐ 3. Current prescription medications.
- ☐ 4. Degree of medications compliance.
- ☐ 5. The children's reaction to their father.
- ☐ 6. Inquiry into the client's recent weight loss.
- ☐ 7. Questions about the vacation itinerary.
- ☐ 8. Questions about financial stability.
- ☐ 9. The client's opinion about what previously occurred psychiatrically.
- ☐ 10. The client's fallback plans should he experience any further compromise.

NOW GO TO SECTION D.

Section C: Diagnostic Relevance of Secondary Information Explored.

1. Administration of the Folstein Mini-Mental Status Examination.
INDICATED (+2)

The Folstein Mini-Mental Status Examination is a well-validated way to cursorily review a client's overall mental functioning, as well as testing a client's orientation to person, place, and time, registration (the capacity to receive and respond to verbal prompts), attention and calculation, memory, language capacity, repetition (reciting a given phrase), and the capacity to follow multi-step commands. It does not, however, adequately evaluate executive functioning (planning, organizing, strategizing, and managing details, time and space), judgment or insight, among other things. However, some sense of this can typically be derived in the course of a reasonably in-depth conversation. In this case, the client scored 30 of 30 on the exam, and was able to follow and attend to all questions and provide reasonably well-considered responses. No evidence of cognitive compromise was noted. Groom and hygiene also appeared to be appropriate, and there were no signs of agitation, pressured speech, attention to internal stimuli, or other signs of psychosis.

2. Direct questions about substance abuse.
INDICATED (+2)

The client denied any past history of illicit substance abuse. Although the ex-wife's prior statements were compelling and detailed, no further evidence to support this concern was obtained from the client.

3. Current prescription medications.
INDICATED (+2)

The client acknowledges having recently taken prescription muscle relaxant medications for a back strain, but denies taking any during the time he was driving or with the children. He states that he has no other prescription medications at this time.

4. Degree of medications compliance.
NOT INDICATED (-1)

Given that he has no active medications prescribed, this would not be indicated.

5. The children's reaction to their father.
INDICATED (+2)

The reaction of the children to their father was entirely within normal limits. The children seemed relaxed and comfortable in his presence, and eager for the latter part of their vacation to begin.

6. Inquiry into the client's recent weight loss.
INDICATED (+1)

The client indicated that he has made a deliberate effort to lose weight since becoming involved with a new romantic interest. He denies taking any medications to accomplish this, and seems to be at a reasonably appropriate weight for his height and build.

7. Questions about the vacation itinerary.
INDICATED (+1)

Non-custodial parents are typically not permitted to take children out of state without written permission from the custodial parent. Further, issues of safety (e.g., hours and duration of driving, etc.) can be considered by such a discussion. The father's itinerary presented as reasonable and safe for the period involved, and he was not crossing state lines.

8. Questions about financial stability.
NOT INDICATED (-1)

This would not be of significance in this situation. The father is well employed, and presents as having ample funds for his needs (e.g., well dressed, driving a newer model car, meeting child support and alimony obligations in a timely way, etc.).

9. The client's opinion about what previously occurred psychiatrically.
INDICATED (+2)

This client showed some signs of agitation when asked about this. He carefully admitted that he had experienced something of a "breakdown," but appeared to minimize the significance of what had happened. When asked for more specific thoughts, he suggested that a "PTSD" event "may have occurred" due to fatigue. He offered no other insight or speculation.

10. The client's fallback plans should he experience any further compromise.
INDICATED (+2)

The client notes that he and the children will be traveling in the same area that his mother lives, and indeed will be spending some time directly with her. Therefore, if he feels compromised in any way, he can always divert to seek her assistance as/if needed.

This page is intentionally blank.

Section D: Provisional Diagnosis Formulation.

Based upon the available information, what would appear to be the most appropriate provisional diagnosis?

DIRECTIONS: Select the most appropriate primary diagnosis indicated in this section. Check your answer. If your answer is not the one indicated write down your point value, then choose another answer and check your score again. Your score from this section will be the numbers added together. (For example: If your first choice was not indicated and had a score of -1, and your second answer choice was the one indicated with a score of +3, your score for this section would be a +2.)

- ☐ 1. Delusional Disorder (F22).
- ☐ 2. Post-Traumatic Stress Disorder (F43.10).
- ☐ 3. Other Psychoactive Substance Use, Unspecified with Psychoactive Substance-induced Psychotic Disorder with Delusions (F19.950).
- ☐ 4. Brief Psychotic Disorder (F23).
- ☐ 5. Malingerer (conscious simulation) (Z76.5).
- ☐ 6. Illness, unspecified (R69).

Section D: Relevance and Diagnostic Formulation.

1. Delusional Disorder (F22).
NOT INDICATED (-1)

This diagnosis is focused on "non-bizarre delusions (i.e., involving situations that occur in real life, such as being followed, poisoned, infected, loved at a distance, or deceived by spouse or lover, or having a disease)." However, it requires that the delusion persist for "at least 1 month's duration." As this client's problems resolved within 48 hours, this would not be an appropriate diagnosis.

2. Post-Traumatic Stress Disorder (F43.10).
NOT INDICATED (-1)

The DSM indicates the diagnosis of PTSD is appropriate "when an individual who has been exposed to a traumatic event develops anxiety symptoms, re-experiencing of the event, and avoidance of stimuli related to the event lasting more than four weeks." The client does have a history of PTSD. Further, some research indicates that PTSD can be comorbid with and even a precursor to psychotic conditions such as delusions. However, as noted in the text, "Novel Approaches to the Diagnosis and Treatment of Posttraumatic Stress Disorder" (2006), PTSD patients typically "retain some reality-testing and insight" during such delusional experiences, and "complex delusions" are "rare in PTSD." Further, the intense persistence of the delusion, apparently for two full days, followed by its complete and total remission, suggests that something else may be involved.

3. Other Psychoactive Substance Use, Unspecified with Psychoactive Substance-induced Psychotic Disorder with Delusions (F19.950).
NOT INDICATED (-1)

While there is considerable circumstantial evidence that the client may be abusing both illicit and prescription drugs, there is no firm evidence of this. Consequently, even though the pattern of delusional thinking and paranoid hallucinations (seeing pursuers in parked cars that were not there) could readily be a result of substance abuse, this diagnosis cannot be properly established.

4. Brief Psychotic Disorder (F23).
INDICATED (+3)

This diagnosis requires that delusional and/or hallucinatory symptoms of psychosis be present for "at least 1 day but less than 1 month, with eventual full return to premorbid level of functioning." The client's presentation properly fits this diagnostic category. Because there is no known precipitating event, entry of the diagnosis should also include the notation, "Without Marked Stressor(s)."

5. Malingerer (conscious simulation) (Z76.5).
NOT INDICATED (-1)

The complexity and persistence of the client's behaviors, even in the face of numerous others, and the fact that no obvious secondary gains were apparent, make this an unlikely diagnosis.

6. Illness, unspecified (R69).
NOT INDICATED (-1)

This diagnosis is entered where insufficient information is available to arrive at an appropriate diagnosis. In the current situation, there is enough diagnostic information (from both the client and others) for a reasonable diagnosis to be made. Therefore, a proper provisional diagnosis can be entered, rather than deferring the diagnosis altogether.

SCORING: (Max = maximum possible; MPL = minimum passing level)

9A. Max 7; MPL 5
9B. Max 8; MPL 6
9C. Max 14; MPL 11
9D. Max 3; MPL 2

This page is intentionally blank.

Simulation #10

The sister of a 26-year-old man, Alex, contacted you upon referral from a former client. She was concerned about the well-being of her brother. He was a graduate student in a doctoral physics program at a major university, and had been doing well academically throughout his undergraduate and graduate studies. Recently, however, he had stopped attending classes, and university staff and friends had begun to call and voice concerns about his increasingly "odd" behavior. By the time she was able to drive out and see Alex, the sister was surprised to find his apartment a jumbled mess. Unwashed clothing was strewn about, half-eaten food containers were everywhere, and spoiled food was in the refrigerator. Old apparently unpaid bills, junk mail, and partially completed homework papers littered the table and floors throughout the apartment. Looking at some of the papers, she could see that his writing often trailed across the pages in nonsensical gibberish. Calculations ran down the sides and backs of the pages and seemed to consist either of circular recapitulation, or else of formulas and mathematical operations only partially completed, over and over again. When she greeted her brother, she found him to be as disheveled as the apartment. His hair was unkempt and his teeth unbrushed, his clothes were smelly and rumpled, and he hadn't shaved in what appeared to be some time. The sister is asking what she should do next.

NOW GO TO SECTION A.

Section A: Initial Information Gathering.

Given the information provided, which of the following would be important in determining the best response?

DIRECTIONS: Select as many as you consider correct. After making your selections and scoring your answers, it is beneficial to read the rationales and extended scenarios for all answer choices.

- ☐ 1. Client's communication patterns and responses to others.
- ☐ 2. Interpersonal relationships/support systems.
- ☐ 3. Duration and intensity of psychiatric symptoms.
- ☐ 4. Past academic performance (grades).
- ☐ 5. Medical history.
- ☐ 6. Psychiatric history.
- ☐ 7. Substance abuse history.
- ☐ 8. Mood status.
- ☐ 9. Vocational/employment history.
- ☐ 10. Collateral contact information.
- ☐ 11. Legal history.
- ☐ 12. Safety issues (driving, firearms, intent to harm self/others, etc.).

NOW GO TO SECTION B.

Section A: Relevance and Initial Information Obtained.

1. Client's communication patterns and responses to others.
INDICATED (+2)

The sister described the client as reluctant to speak with others, and talking in ways that did not seem to make sense. For example, he said he had stopped going to his classes because the professors were telling other students "bad things" about him. He wasn't able to finish most meals, because he would discover "poison had been put in the food" even before the meal was done—he suspected people were sneaking in during his meals and putting the poison in when he wasn't looking. He had turned off his heating unit, even though there was snow outside, because he had discovered that the unit was a "conduit" that was used to "draw spirits inside the house" that would trouble him night and day. If he kept the unit turned off, he could keep most of the spirits away.

2. Interpersonal relationships/support systems.
NOT INDICATED (-1)

This information may be helpful in determining resources and sources of support to help the client, but it would not be directly useful in determining a best response to his immediate presentation.

3. Duration and intensity of psychiatric symptoms.
INDICATED (+2)

In explaining the "spirits" that troubled him, the client explained that they were "like shadows" most of the time, but that he could see them sometimes, if he was watchful enough. Then, he added that he could "hear them" almost all of the time, even if he couldn't see them, and they often pushed him to "do things." Asked what things they might tell him, he explained that it was "just different things." Then, displaying a healed cut on his left forearm, he indicated that he had once been told to "cut his arm and drain out some poison" that he had "accidentally eaten" with his meals. When he did, he felt much better. The client indicated that the problems had been "getting worse for a couple of months," but that once he had stopped going to classes and running the heat in his apartment, things were "a little better." When asked about the piles of papers, notes, homework exercises, and calculations all over the house, the client explained that he had found "special codes" in his textbooks, and he was trying to decipher the messages—especially those that would help him to keep the troubling spirits away.

4. Past academic performance (grades).
NOT INDICATED (-2)

Not immediately relevant to the client's situation.

5. Medical history.
INDICATED (+1)

The client had no remarkable past medical history and was not then under a physician's care; nor was he taking any prescription or over the counter medications.

6. Psychiatric history.

INDICATED (+2)

Per the sister, the client had no prior psychiatric history. She felt he was somewhat prone to becoming "stressed out" when under pressure, and she speculated that his winter term final examinations may have overwhelmed him in some way. She denied any knowledge of the client having experienced major depression, grandiosity or mania, or other episodes of psychosis in the past.

7. Substance abuse history.

INDICATED (+1)

The sister indicated that she knew of no such history, but could not be certain as she had married and moved away when the client was still in high school.

8. Mood status.

INDICATED (+2)

The sister described the client's mood as agitated, suspicious, and anxious.

9. Vocational/employment history.

NOT INDICATED (-1)

Vocational and employment history is not relevant in formulating a response to the client's current situation. However, the client's education was being paid for out of a substantial "trust fund" left by their deceased parents. Consequently, the client had no prior employment history as he had been a student virtually continuously since graduation from high school.

10. Collateral contact information.

INDICATED (+2)

The sister was the client's only living immediate family. The parents were deceased (the last, approximately two years previously), and they were the only children. Other contacts, however, included campus professors and the client's classmates. In inquiring further, it was learned that the client had remained aloof from others for the most part, but he had been generally communicative with his doctoral advisor and certain key classmates. These individuals suggested that his "problems" had begun about two months into the current term. He had started to neglect his appearance and had begun missing classes. Eventually, he was avoiding all efforts to communicate. When campus staff and others could no longer reach him, they placed the call of concern to his sister.

11. Legal history.

NOT INDICATED (-1)

This would not be specifically germane to the client's immediate situation, although it could prove helpful later. However, the sister indicated that he had no legal history of which she was aware.

12. Safety issues (driving, firearms, intent to harm self/others, etc.).
INDICATED (+3)

The client lived in student housing adjacent to the campus. Therefore, he had no car, as he could meet all shopping and other needs either on foot or on the bicycle that he kept in his apartment. In addition, he had no firearm, and had expressed no specific intent to harm himself or others. He had, however, cut himself some two weeks previously, in response to some form of command auditory hallucination.

RESPONSE FORMULATION:

The client was suffering from obvious symptoms of psychosis. The duration of symptoms was longer than one month. There was no immediate evidence of bipolar disorder (manic and/or depressive symptoms), nor was there evidence of substance abuse. Although the client had not been medically evaluated recently, all indications were that he had been healthy up to this point. He was not under a doctor's care, and was not taking any prescription or over-the-counter medications. Per the sister, he was also not taking any vitamin supplements or herbal preparations of any kind. Therefore, it was unlikely that a medical condition was responsible for his current presentation. The client had, however, been under considerable stress with his doctoral studies and recent final examinations. Over the last 2-3 months, he had deteriorated in his hygiene and grooming, and appeared unable to manage ordinary standards of cleanliness of his home and person. He had been experiencing both auditory and visual hallucinations, and appeared to be suffering from delusions as well. The client had also experienced at least one episode of "command auditory hallucinations" that resulted in self-injury. Further, he had cut off his heating during a period of substantial cold, and had not been eating properly. Finally, his confusion and/or avolition had progressed to the point that he had many unpaid bills, suggesting that he would be at further risk of losing phone service, electricity, and other necessary utilities and services.

Section B: Based on the intake data available, identify the most appropriate response.

DIRECTIONS: Select the most effective option available. Check your answer. If your answer is not the IDEAL option, write down your point value, then choose another answer and check your score again. Your score from this section will be the numbers added together. (For example: If your first choice was not indicated and had a score of -1, and your second answer choice was the one indicated with a score of +3, your score for this section would be a +2.)

- ☐ 1. Have the sister call the police.
- ☐ 2. Refer the sister to a "crisis hotline."
- ☐ 3. Direct the sister to the local Adult Protective Services program.
- ☐ 4. Recommend the sister take the client to a local hospital.
- ☐ 5. Suggest an immediate office visit for further evaluation.
- ☐ 6. Tell the sister to monitor the situation and call if things worsen.

NOW GO TO SECTION C.

Section B: Relevance of Potential Response Options.

1. Have the sister call the police.
NOT RECOMMENDED (-1)

Law enforcement can do a good job of managing psychiatric disturbances. However, they are most properly called "in the line of duty"—to manage misconduct, violent, and/or criminal behavior—rather than for evaluative purposes. Indeed, they may be reluctant to dispatch for a complaint such as this, particularly if other demands have precluded these services.

2. Refer the sister to a "crisis hotline."
NOT RECOMMENDED (-1)

"Crisis hotlines" are normally for situations if imminent disaster or compromise—suicide, toxic overdose, etc.—as opposed to gradually unfolding problems.

3. Direct the sister to the local Adult Protective Services program.
GOOD OPTION (+1)

Referral to a local Adult Protection Services program is a good referral option. They are well-equipped to evaluate such situations, and may even be the ideal option in many situations (e.g., when someone needs to be immediately removed from an abusive or dangerous situation, etc.). However, these programs are often over-utilized and under-funded. They struggle to meet the demands placed upon them. Therefore, all other reasonable options should be explored before this referral is made.

4. Recommend the sister take the client to a local hospital.
ACCEPTABLE OPTION (0)

The client is clearly compromised psychiatrically, and many large medical facilities will have psychiatric resources. If the client is insured and has a primary care provider, taking the client to be seen medically is one option—and one that will likely become necessary at some point in the evaluative process. However, primary care providers have extremely limited time to spend with any one patient (7-14 minutes, on average), and thus, the visit will likely only result in another appointment with a specialist—often at some significant delay. Thus, other reasonable options should be explored before this option is selected.

5. Suggest an immediate office visit for further evaluation.
IDEAL OPTION (+3)

This would be the ideal first option in this situation. It offers several advantages. First, the clinical office is often far less threatening to confused clients than a large medical center, or confronting law enforcement, etc. Second, you are already becoming well informed about the client's situation, and thus, better equipped to facilitate the intake and engagement process compared with having the family recapitulate the entire story with someone new. Third, the clinical encounter is usually longer and therefore, more productive in this setting. Fourth, necessary referrals and further evaluation for needed medications can often be expedited via an existing clinician-psychiatrist professional relationship.

6. Tell the sister to monitor the situation and call if things worsen.
DANGEROUS (-2)

This client has already inflicted minor self-harm in response to some form of "command" auditory hallucination and/or delusion. Further, his cognitive integrity is rapidly decompensating, and his home situation is becoming further compromised and even dangerous. Therefore, it is crucial that something be done promptly.

ADDITIONAL INFORMATION: The sister prevailed upon Alex to come and see you, under the guise of "getting help to keep the troubling spirits away." Upon meeting the client, you noted his continued disheveled appearance, poor hygiene and grooming, and his marked preoccupation with internal stimuli. He refused to answer most mental status questions, and so, completion of a Mental Status Exam was not possible at that time. However, his presentation offered considerable information. For example, he often took considerable time before responding to you, as if attending to internal stimuli. Further, his affect was routinely not congruent with speech content—with verbalized expressions of laughter, suspicion, anger, and other emotive states arising without provocation or context. At times, he was muttering to himself, responding to questions and comments solely within his own mind. His speech was frequently pressured and anxious, and his thoughts were often marked by dyslogia—specifically, paralogia (illogical or delusional thoughts)—and dereism, tangentiality, derailment, and flights of fantasy. Ideas of reference were also apparent as he presumed, for example, that a brief telephone call received by the secretary was actually about him and his situation, etc., when it was clearly just the confirmation of another client's appointment. Even so, he was very interested in receiving help to better cope with the "troubling spirits," and therefore, was willing to cooperate with an early treatment plan.

This page is intentionally blank.

Section C: Provisional Diagnosis Formulation

Based on the available information, what would appear to be the most appropriate provisional diagnosis?

DIRECTIONS: Select the most appropriate provisional diagnosis indicated in this section. Check your answer. If your answer is not the one indicated write down your point value, then choose another answer and check your score again. Your score from this section will be the numbers added together. (For example: If your first choice was not indicated and had a score of -1, and your second answer choice was the one indicated with a score of +3, your score for this section would be a +2.)

- ☐ 1. Delusional Disorder (F22).
- ☐ 2. Schizotypal Disorder (F21).
- ☐ 3. Schizophrenia, unspecified (F20.9)
- ☐ 4. Schizoaffective Disorder, unspecified (F25.9).
- ☐ 5. Brief Psychotic Disorder (F23).
- ☐ 6. Other Schizophrenia (F20.89).
- ☐ 7. Schizophreniform Disorder (F20.81).

NOW GO TO SECTION D.

Section C: Potential Relevance and Diagnostic Formulation

1. Delusional Disorder (F22).
NOT INDICATED (-1)

The diagnosis of delusional disorder is partially met, but as the client is obviously having delusions along with hallucinations which makes the clients situation not meet criteria B. Also his life's functioning is obviously very impaired and bizarre.

2. Schizotypal Disorder (F21).
NOT INDICATED (-1)

The criteria for this disorder are not met as the symptoms have so far only been met during the course of schizophrenia or another psychotic disorder (schizophreniform disorder). Also, personality disorders should not be diagnosed in one visit but multiple visits and information gathering.

3. Schizophrenia, unspecified (F20.9)
NOT INDICATED (-1)

Given the client's marked delusions, hallucinations, and disorganized speech and behavior, a diagnosis of schizophrenia would be anticipated. However, a diagnosis of schizophrenia is only made when the disturbance has persisted "for at least 6 months," and this client has only been symptomatic for 2-3 months, per available reports.

4. Schizoaffective Disorder, unspecified (F25.9).
NOT INDICATED (-1)

In schizoaffective disorder, there are symptoms of a mood disorder during the symptoms of schizophrenia. However, as of so far, no mood symptoms are being reported for this client.

5. Brief Psychotic Disorder (F23).
NOT INDICATED (-1)

The client has been symptomatic for 2-3 months, per available reports, and a diagnosis of Brief Psychotic Disorder can only be made when symptoms have been present for less than a month and have resolved completely. Therefore, this would not be an appropriate diagnosis.

6. Other Schizophrenia (F20.89)
NOT INDICATED (-1)

This diagnosis would only be used where no other appropriate diagnosis is available. In the case of this client, a more definitive diagnosis is available.

7. Schizophreniform Disorder (F20.81).
INDICATED (+3)

This category is used when a client has met all diagnostic criteria for schizophrenia in Categories A, D, and E, but when the condition resolves within one to six months. Where the diagnosis is applied prior to recovery, it must be qualified as "provisional." This fits the client's clinical presentation at present. Because of the slow and insidious nature of onset (over a period of more than four weeks, per reports), and because of the client's preexisting limited social and occupational functioning, a qualifier of "Without Good Prognostic Features" may be appropriate.

This page is intentionally blank.

Section D: Treatment Planning.

DIRECTIONS: Select from this section, the single most appropriate early treatment option that you can provide. Check your answer. If your answer is not the one indicated write down your point value, then choose another answer and check your score again. Your score from this section will be the numbers added together. (For example: If your first choice was not indicated and had a score of -1, and your second answer choice was the one indicated with a score of +3, your score for this section would be a +2.)

- ☐ 1. Cognitive-behavioral therapy.
- ☐ 2. Psychiatric hospitalization.
- ☐ 3. Relaxation and imagery techniques.
- ☐ 4. Reality therapy.
- ☐ 5. Psychiatrist referral for antipsychotic medications.
- ☐ 6. Group therapy.

NOW GO TO SECTION E.

Section D: Early Treatment Options—Relevance and Findings.

1. Cognitive-behavioral therapy.
NOT INDICATED (-1)

This approach can be helpful later on, particularly in helping an individual with medication compliance. However, early on when symptoms of psychosis are still evident, it is not a productive approach. It can even be counter-productive in cases of more severe psychosis.

2. Psychiatric hospitalization.
NOT INDICATED (-1)

Given that antipsychotic medications can usually reduce psychotic symptoms very quickly, hospitalization is unlikely to be necessary. Only in situations of refractory treatment or uncertain safety would this be considered an "early" intervention.

3. Relaxation and imagery techniques.
NOT INDICATED (-1)

While relaxation and imagery techniques can be effective in many situations, such techniques are not generally effective with individuals experiencing psychotic symptoms.

4. Reality therapy.
NOT INDICATED (-1)

As with cognitive-behavioral therapy, this would not be considered an "early" treatment approach, because the symptoms of psychosis typically preclude rational thinking.

5. Psychiatrist referral for antipsychotic medications.
INDICATED (+3)

This would be the treatment of immediate choice. Antipsychotic medications can provide profound relief from troubling psychotic symptoms, and can then make way for other collateral treatments of further value and support.

6. Group therapy.
NOT INDICATED (-1)

While group therapy can be especially valuable once an individual's symptoms of psychosis have been controlled, it is not an effective treatment for individuals suffering with the hallucinations, delusions, confusion, and anxious and paranoid features common to untreated schizophrenia.

ADDITIONAL INFORMATION: Over the next six months, you continue to follow and monitor the client's progress. The antipsychotic medication provided (Haldol, a.k.a., haloperidol) has been effective, and the client's delusions and hallucinations now appear to be greatly improved. They are not, however, entirely absent and readily reemerge if his medications are titrated down. Therefore, his diagnosis has now been formalized as Schizophrenia (F20.9). However, during the last few visits, you note that the client has begun to express distress over a marked sense of physical restlessness. Specifically, he seems to be having trouble remaining still. These early "Extrapyramidal Side Effects" (EPS) are common when individuals are started on a regimen of antipsychotic medications (i.e., neuroleptics) and may become permanent, especially if left untreated. His symptoms include: 1) restless movements (rocking from one foot to another), 2) walking on the spot, 3) shuffling and swinging one leg on the other while sitting, and 4) pacing even when he would like to stop. Symptoms of this nature occur in as many as 49% of patients treated with typical antipsychotics. Improperly diagnosed, the symptoms could be mistaken for worsening of psychotic symptoms, erroneously leading to a higher dose of the neuroleptic, further exacerbating the problem.

This page is intentionally blank.

Section E: Based on the above information, identify the appropriate term for the client's extrapyramidal symptoms.

DIRECTIONS: Select the appropriate term from among the following. Check your answer. If your answer is not the one indicated write down your point value, then choose another answer and check your score again. Your score from this section will be the numbers added together. (For example: If your first choice was not indicated and had a score of -1, and your second answer choice was the one indicated with a score of +3, your score for this section would be a +2.)

- ☐ 1. Drug-induced Parkinsonism.
- ☐ 2. Chorea.
- ☐ 3. Athetosis.
- ☐ 4. Akathisia.
- ☐ 5. Choreoathetosis.
- ☐ 6. Tardive Dyskinesia.

NOW GO TO SECTION F.

Section E: Term and description of the conditions.

1. Drug-induced Parkinsonism.
NOT CORRECT (-1)

The triad of resting tremor, muscular rigidity, and bradykinesia characterizes neuroleptic-induced Parkinsonism. The symptoms of tremor may involve other muscles, such as those of the lips and perioral muscles, which may produce a rabbit-like movement of the face. The muscular rigidity varies. It may present as a "lead-pipe" (constant resistance) type or a "cogwheel" type (when a tremor coexists with rigidity, producing a rhythmic, intermittent resistance). Bradykinesia is evident in a mask-like facial expression, difficulty initiating movement, or in reduced accessory limb movement. Symptoms usually manifest within 3 months of the onset of drug therapy.

2. Chorea.
NOT CORRECT (-1)

The ad hoc Committee on Classification of the World Federation of Neurology has defined chorea as "a state of excessive, spontaneous movements, irregularly timed, non-repetitive, randomly distributed and abrupt in character. These movements may vary in severity from restlessness with mild intermittent exaggeration of gesture and expression, fidgeting movements of the hands, unstable dance-like gait to a continuous flow of disabling, violent movements."

Individuals with chorea present with 1) motor impersistence (i.e., an inability to maintain a sustained posture); 2) difficulty gripping objects (they alternately squeeze and release, called "milkmaid's grip," causing them to frequently drop things); and 3) when asked to protrude the tongue, it tends to pop in and out (called "harlequin's tongue"). Individuals may attempt to mask the chorea by deliberately imposing semi-purposeful movements over the choreiform movements.

3. Athetosis.
NOT CORRECT (-1)

This is a slow form of chorea. Because of the slowness, the movements have a writhing (i.e., squirming, twisting, or snakelike) appearance. The writhing movements are extremely prominent, even apart from the speed of the movement. Therefore, the authors of this article advocate retaining this descriptive term.

4. Akathisia.
CORRECT (+3)

This condition involves a subjective feeling of restlessness, often progressing to overt signs of restlessness. Restless movements, such as rocking, walking in place, shuffling and pacing are common symptoms. The individual feels great distress, as the drive to move cannot be controlled, and may lead to considerable fatigue. This apparent "agitation" may also erroneously lead to an inappropriate escalation in the neuroleptic dose, inadvertently worsening the problem.

5. Choreoathetosis.
NOT CORRECT (-1)

Choreoathetoid movements are essentially an intermediate form between chorea and athetosis—slower than chorea and faster than typical athetosis. These movements may manifest in the same individual at different times, or in different body extremities. This term underscores the point that the primary difference between chorea, choreoathetosis, and athetosis is the speed of the movements involved.

6. Tardive Dyskinesia.
NOT CORRECT (-1)

A syndrome of persistent involuntary hyperkinetic abnormal movements that most frequently occur in the face (tongue thrusting, chewing, side to side or rotary jaw movements, lip smacking, rapid eye blinking), but also may involve uncontrolled and purposeless movements in the limbs and trunk. It occurs in 15-20% of predisposed patients. It typically has a delayed onset that is associated with long-term treatment with neuroleptics.

This page is intentionally blank.

Section F: Identify the most effective therapeutic approaches for use in treating the client's extrapyramidal symptoms.

DIRECTIONS: Select the most appropriate therapeutic approach(es) in this section. After making your selections and scoring your answers, it is beneficial to read the rationales and extended scenarios for all answer choices.

- ☐ 1. Reducing the neuroleptic dose.
- ☐ 2. Switching to a medication with a lower EPS profile.
- ☐ 3. The addition of anticholinergic drugs to overcome EPS symptoms.
- ☐ 4. The addition of a benzodiazepine or beta-blocker.

Section F: Element Relevance and Commentary.

1. Reducing the neuroleptic dose.
INDICATED (+1)

This therapeutic approach is not always possible when break-through symptoms of psychosis occur, but can be effective in some cases.

2. Switching to a medication with a lower EPS profile.
INDICATED (+2)

Newer atypical antipsychotic medications, such as such as aripiprazole, ziprasidone, quetiapine, olanzapine, risperidone, or clozapine, are less likely to induce or maintain EPS symptoms.

3. The addition of anticholinergic drugs to overcome EPS symptoms.
INDICATED (+1)

Anticholinergic and antihistaminergic medications. Trihexyphenidyl (2 to 8 mg per day) and benztropine (2 to 8 mg per day) are among the most common anticholinergics given.

4. The addition of a benzodiazepine or beta-blocker.
INDICATED (+1)

This approach is more appropriate for self-esteem issues, situational disorders, etc., but it is not optimally effective in treating panic disorder.

SCORING: (Max = maximum possible; MPL = minimum passing level)

10A. Max 15; MPL 11
10B. Max 4; MPL 3
10C. Max 3; MPL 2
10D. Max 3; MPL 2
10E. Max 3; MPL 2
10F. Max 5; MPL 4

Thank You

We at Mometrix would like to extend our heartfelt thanks to you, our friend and patron, for allowing us to play a part in your journey. It is a privilege to serve people from all walks of life who are unified in their commitment to building the best future they can for themselves.

The preparation you devote to these important testing milestones may be the most valuable educational opportunity you have for making a real difference in your life. We encourage you to put your heart into it—that feeling of succeeding, overcoming, and yes, conquering will be well worth the hours you've invested.

We want to hear your story, your struggles and your successes, and if you see any opportunities for us to improve our materials so we can help others even more effectively in the future, please share that with us as well. **The team at Mometrix would be absolutely thrilled to hear from you!** So please, send us an email (support@mometrix.com) and let's stay in touch.

If you feel as though you need additional help, please check out the other resources we offer:

Study Guide: http://MometrixStudyGuides.com/NCMHCE

Flashcards: http://MometrixFlashcards.com/NCMHCE